THE NATURAL MEDICINE GUIDE FOR TRAVEL & HOME

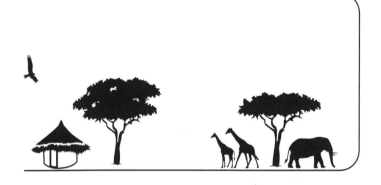

RICHARD PITT

IMPORTANT NOTICE

Medicine, like every other science, is subject to continuous development. Research and clinical experience broaden our knowledge, particularly as far as treatment and medical therapy are concerned. Whenever there are dosages or applications mentioned in this manual, the reader may rest assured that the author, editor and publishers have taken great care to ensure that the information given represents the standard of knowledge at the time of completion of this book.

The information in this book reflects the experience and study of the author and the information on all the remedies mentioned is widely available in standard homeopathic medical texts and other natural medicine books. However, the accuracy and effectiveness of any of the recommendations made in the book cannot be guaranteed and this book is not intended to replace professional medical care in situations where that is required. The book is designed to be used as a guide in aiding self-treatment and not as the only source of information about the given subject matter. Therefore, the authors, editors and publishers cannot make any promise of the effectiveness of any of the treatments mentioned. Readers are suggested to also consult other material and references on the subject and to consult a medical professional if indicated.

The recommended dosages and any possible contraindications are general recommendations and therefore are used at the reader's own risk. However, the authors and publishers appeal to each user to pass on any pertinent information of any reaction that comes to his or her notice.

The author and publisher cannot accept any liability for any loss or damage caused by the content of this book and make no warranties about the effectiveness of any suggested treatment. However, it is hoped that the information is of practical use to all who read the book.

Protected trade names (trademarks) are not marked in any special way. Therefore, it should not be assumed from the lack of such a mark that the trade name is free.

All rights to this manual including all or any of its parts are reserved. Any use of this manual or parts thereof outside the narrow confines of the copyright law without prior permission of the publishers is prohibited and will be prosecuted. This applies in particular to photocopies, translations, microfilms and storage and processing in electronic systems.

Title	The Natural Medicine Guide For Travel and Home
	www.thenaturalmedicineguide.com
Author	Richard Pitt
ISBN/EAN	978-94-90453-08-4
Edition	1st Edition
Cover design	13² Studio San Francisco, California
Lay–out	13² Studio San Francisco, California
Editor	Jenni Tree
Publisher	Homeolinks Publishers
	P.O. Box 68, 9750 AB Haren, Netherlands
	E office@homeolinks.nl
	Website www.homeolinks.nl
Printer	CreateSpace

THE NATURAL MEDICINE GUIDE FOR TRAVEL & HOME

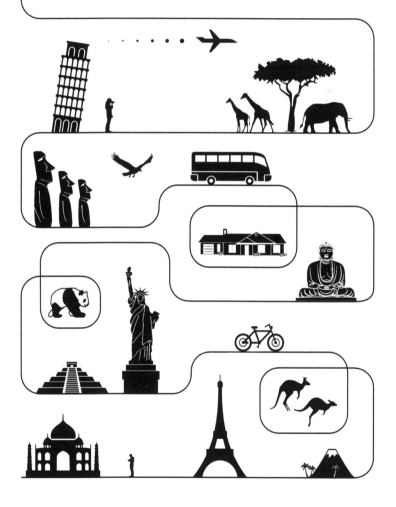

RICHARD PITT

Acknowledgements

It has been said it takes a village to raise a child. Bringing a book to fruition is not much different. You think it's a good idea, you carry the vision, begin the writing process and then at a certain time, you look around for help. Books can take a huge amount of effort to write and quite impossible without the help of many people. So I would like to thank everybody who helped me with this book; from friends who put me up all over the world while I 'write', to others who gave comments and advice on the book; to colleagues in the field of homeopathy who I have worked with over the years and to friends and family who have supported me in so many ways and simply being there when it was needed. Thank you to one and all.

Contents

Foreword		ix
Preface		xi
Introduction		xiii
One The Foundations of Natural Medicine		1
Two How to use Natural Medicines		15
Three Being Prepared		21
Four Accidents, Injuries and Trauma		33
Accidents and injury		33
Altitude sickness		36
Bites		37
Burns		37
Concussion		43
Emergencies and Disasters		46
Fainting		48
Fractures		48
Frostbite		49
Hangover		50
Headache		50
Heatstroke		51
Hemorrhage		52
Jetlag		53
Pain		54
Poisoning		55
Shock		56
Sleeplessness		58
Spinal injury		60
Sprains		60
Surgery		61
Travel sickness		62
Wounds		62

Five Emotional conditions   **65**

Anger 65
Anxiety 66
Fright 67
Grief 68

Six Digestive conditions   **71**

Abdominal pain 71
Appendicitis 71
Colic 73
Constipation 74
Diaper rash 75
Diarrhea 75
Dysentery 79
Food poisoning 82
Hemorrhoids 83
Hepatitis 84
Indigestion 87
Nausea 89
Worms 89

Seven Common Infections   **93**

Simple fever 93
Influenza 96
Common Children's diseases 100
Chicken pox 101
German measles 102
Measles 103
Mumps 103
Whooping cough. 104

Eight Colds and Coughs   **107**

Colds 107
Coughs (including bronchitis and pneumonia) 108

Nine ENT: Ear, (Eyes, Mouth), Nose and Throat   **113**

Allergies 113
Cold sores (Herpes) 115
Ear pain 116
Injury to the Ear 118
Eye conditions: Inflammations 118
Blepharitis 118
Conjunctivitis 118

Styes and Chalazae 119
Injury to the Eye 120
Mouth ulcers 120
Sinusitis 121
Teething 122
Throat conditions 123
Toothache 124

Ten Women's conditions   **127**
Breast conditions 127
Pregnancy and Birth 129
Nausea 130
Miscarriage 131
Labor 132
After birth 133

Eleven Bladder and Kidneys   **135**
Cystitis 135
Kidney disease 137

Twelve Skin conditions   **139**
Animals (bedbugs, lice, fleas) 140
Boils 141
Chilblains 143
Fungal infections 143
Hives 145
Impetigo 146
Poison oak/ivy 147
Scabies 148
Shingles 149
Ulcers 150

Thirteen Common Tropical diseases   **153**
Dengue Fever 153
Malaria 155
Typhoid 162

Fourteen Other Tropical and infectious diseases   **167**
African Sleeping Sickness 174
Bilharzia/Schistosomiasis 175
Brucellosis 177
Chagas Disease 178
Cholera 179

Diphtheria 181
Filiariasis 181
Guinea worm 182
Hookworm disease 183
Japanese Encephalitis 184
Lassa Fever 185
Leishmaniasis 186
Leptospirosis 188
Plague 189
Poliomyelitis 190
Rabies 191
Rift Valley Fever 192
Trachoma 193
West Nile Virus 193
Yellow Fever 194

Fifteen Tick bite diseases   **197**
Lyme Disease 197
Colorado Tick Fever 202
European Tick Borne Encephalitis 202
Relapsing Fever 203
Rocky Mountain Spotted Fever 204

Sixteen Prevention   **205**
The Three Main Types of Travel 207
Immunizations and Natural Prevention 208
Vaccine Risks and Benefits 212
The Main Travel Vaccines and Prevention Methods 213

Seventeen Homeopathic and Herbal remedy list   **239**
Homeopathic Remedies 239
Herbal remedies and Essential Oils 267

Eighteen Resources and References   **273**

Index of Conditions   **279**

Foreword

If, like Richard you enjoy traveling roads less traveled and visiting places where you can have a real taste of a country, its people and their culture, then having a travel companion to guard your health and well being is more than welcome. This Natural Medicine Guide is the kind of companion that can follow you everywhere you go and – if not traveling – should be easily accessible on a kitchen shelf or in a bathroom cupboard.

Richard is passionate about traveling as well as natural medicine. Together with his aptitude for writing this makes him the perfect author for this book. Besides drawing from direct experience based on years of traveling the globe and decades of treating patients with homeopathy, being an avid reader he has also integrated tips from a wealth of sources making this book a rather complete guide for travel and home, covering a wide range of topics. As a traveler you can encounter many situations concerning your health. You name it and you'll find it discussed in this book.

The layout of the book is such that you can easily find the information you need for a specific situation. As making a diagnosis is not something you can always easily do yourself, the book offers you the possibility to nevertheless find a remedy to help by focusing on your main symptoms and looking for remedies there. Then by reading the suggested remedies in the back of the book you can decide what the best choice is for you based on your symptoms.

Do not just buy the book and stick it with your passport. In the guide you will find several recommendations as to what to take with you on your travels so do read it while still at home so you can also benefit from it there and are prepared once you do leave for your next destination.

Even if you're traveling without any need to consult this book – which, being quite a traveler myself, I truly wish for you – then this book is still a great companion. While waiting on a crowded airport or at a dusty bus stop you can have an interesting introduction to natural medicine and the philosophy behind it. It also offers knowledge of how you may be able to help fellow travelers you meet while on the road, even if you are fine yourself. Isn't it great to find out that you brought this guide all the way to help him or her?

Do grant yourself, your family members and travel companions, and those you meet on the road this practical and useful guide.

I wish you happy and healthy travels.

Harry van der Zee MD

Preface

I began to travel seriously after leaving school at age eighteen, spending four years 'on the road' between the UK and Australia, most of the time in Asia and especially India. At that time, India was a challenging place to travel in and it was very common to catch some potentially nasty stomach bugs leading to diarrhea, dysentery and worse. Hepatitis A was very common and if unlucky, malaria, typhoid and dengue fever were not unusual. Luckily I survived it fairly intact, a couple of bouts of intense diarrhea being the worst symptoms I experienced. I did get a mild dose of Hepatitis A, turning yellow with jaundice when arriving home, but I soon recovered and since then all my travels have been fairly incident free. More recently I have spent over one year in Africa, both in West Africa and also in Malawi and Kenya. Africa has some of the nastiest diseases for the traveler to avoid, malaria being by far the most common and one of the worst. Unfortunately I did catch malaria – one bad night in a fishing village on Lake Malawi with a dysfunctional net – but I have recovered well. My experiences in traveling have made me aware of many of the challenges one can face when traveling and also simply living in your home town. This book comes out of this experience.

I did not even know about homeopathy when I was first traveling but soon after returning from my first four years of traveling at age twenty two, I began to study homeopathy seriously. I was inspired by its philosophy and through my travels and studying of world culture and philosophies, the principles of homeopathy and natural medicine made a lot of sense to me. In recognizing the healing power of nature and understanding the concept of the interconnectedness between mind and body and one's environment, the foundations of homeopathic theory connected with me and I thought that if these ideas and principles can be applied directly in the practice of medicine, they must have huge potential. Thirty years later, my experience has confirmed this initial inspiration. I have seen amazing results, both in chronic long term diseases in my practice and also working in the field in Africa and India. I have seen people who are writhing in pain in front of me get better in a matter of minutes when the right remedy is given. This is not an uncommon experience. It has given me the confidence to be able to recommend homeopathy and natural medicine for a wide variety of conditions that anybody can come across.

I have been practicing homeopathy now for over thirty years, initially in England and then in the United States. Although most of this work has been treating chronic conditions found in western cultures, I have also treated many infectious, acute conditions. From over eight years of travel in most parts of the world, I have had the opportunity to use homeopathy in many acute conditions not often seen in the west. I have worked with local people and have helped establish schools and teaching programs for people to learn the fundamentals of homeopathic practice and have also studied homeopathy and spent time with homeopathic practitioners in Greece, India, Australia, New Zealand, Brazil, Africa, Europe and North America. This book is a result of my own experience of practicing homeopathy and of traveling extensively over many years. Most of the natural health options discussed in the book are therefore homeopathic remedies, which can be bought in convenient kits for travel and for storage at home, as well as some important herbal medicine options to complement the homeopathic suggestions. Hopefully this information will give confidence to travel far and wide, knowing that many possible health issues can be addressed effectively. The information in this book can add to your arsenal of health options, both away from home and also for basic day-to-day health issues.

Introduction

The purpose of this book is to give clear and simple options that homeopathy and other natural medicines have to offer for a wide variety of acute conditions. These are particularly relevant at times when traveling and also for first aid use in the home. However, I felt the need also to include situations which are potentially more serious, especially when traveling in challenging areas. Given the limitations of conventional medicine and access to appropriate medical care, especially in more remote places, knowledge of how to treat many simple and some complex health issues is as important today as ever. Homeopathic medicine especially has a good track record in treating many of the conditions mentioned in this book.

The success of homeopathy was clearly documented, first in Europe in the 1820's and 1830's during cholera and typhoid epidemics, as well as in the United States during the deadly flu pandemic of 1918, where statistics showed that homeopaths had a death rate of only 1.05%, in comparison with over 30% under allopathic care, and even up to 60% at times. In the 1st World War in the United States there was a homeopathic medical corps, staffed by 100 nurses, 22 physicians and two dentists, nearly all homeopaths. In 1922, President Harding, whose father served as a homeopathic physician in the Civil War, hosted a convention of homeopaths at the White House. In the late 1800's in the United States, there were 22 homeopathic medical schools, 100 homeopathic hospitals and over 1,000 homeopathic pharmacies.

Today, homeopathy still has solutions for numerous epidemic diseases both old and emerging, as well as for many other diseases. This book is designed to give you access to some of this valuable information. The recommendations in the book however, are not designed to take the place of conventional medical care. Homeopathy can be used along with all other forms of medical care, conventional and otherwise. In any situation, the risks need to be weighed up in deciding the best course of action to take. Ideally this book will help you to be able to evaluate these risks and to know what course of action to take.

Homeopathy is a well proven system of medicine that has been practiced all over the world for over two hundred years. There are now professionally trained homeopaths and people seeking homeopathic and other natural medical care in every continent, including Africa, most of Asia, Europe, North and South America, Russia and China. If you would like to look at the developing body of research into homeopathy, you can find it at the Homeopathy Research Institute **www.homeoinst. org**, among other sites. For more information on organizations, please look at Chapter Eighteen which lists various homeopathic organizations and information resources.

The following chapter gives you a brief introduction to the principles and history of homeopathy and also discusses its relation to herbal medicine and natural therapies in general. When using these remedies, it is useful to have some background information about how they work. It is important to state that using homeopathic and herbal medicine does not take the place of conventional care and often both methods may be used at the same time. However, having simple and effective natural methods available can greatly help when health challenges arise. Each condition needs to be looked at carefully and if any condition in the book is potentially serious, recommendations to get a professional opinion or care are given. Two chapters are then given to the practicalities of how to use natural medicines and also in being prepared for travel. Chapter Three, in particular is important, especially for those inexperienced in traveling to developing countries.

The therapeutic chapters begin in Chapter Four with accidents, injuries and trauma and cover most of the accidents and first aid situations one can experience. It also covers some of the specific experiences of travel, including jet lag and travel sickness. These are some of the most commonly experienced traumas when traveling. It is followed by a chapter on the treatment of emotional conditions. This chapter is given priority as homeopathy can very effectively treat emotional conditions and the connection between emotional and physical states is important to understand when using homeopathic remedies. Chapter Six focuses on digestive conditions, which again are some of the most commonly experienced ailments found when traveling. Ideally, many of these conditions can be avoided by taking precautions outlined in Chapter Three, but sometimes one simply can't avoid getting sick. The following chapters after that cover a wide range of conditions including more serious tropical diseases and infections. The book is designed to be both succinct in its approach but detailed enough to cover most diseases that one could come across, not only when traveling, but also at home.

Chapter Sixteen discusses the conventional and alternative forms of prevention available for various diseases. It discusses vaccination options, their risks and potential benefits. Travelers are always recommended to get many vaccines, some of which can have side effects, making it important to be fully informed. This chapter also assesses the potential risks of many diseases by the type of travel undertaken. Not all traveling is the same and therefore the risks of getting certain diseases also vary. It is important that every person traveling knows as much as possible about the types of diseases they could face and what options are available to avoid getting them.

Chapter Seventeen gives a list of all the remedies mentioned in the book and their main symptom picture. This chapter can be used as a reference and complements the information in each chapter. Some remedies are mentioned a lot in many chapters and for many conditions. Having knowledge of the key points for the most popular remedies can greatly help in recognizing when these remedies are needed. This obviously comes with experience, but ideally this book can help in the study of important homeopathic and herbal remedies used.

The last chapter gives information on homeopathic and health resources and where books and remedies can be found. For those wanting to explore the subject more, some of these resources may be useful. I hope this book helps you in your knowledge of how to use homeopathic and herbal medicines and gives you confidence to use them, wherever you are in the world and in whatever circumstances you are in.

Chapter One
The Foundations of Natural Medicine

Why Natural Medicine?

What does it mean? Using the term 'natural medicine' implies that other forms of medicine are unnatural, which is not exactly correct. It more accurately reflects the distinction between using methods and substances that are taken directly from nature and that work with the body's own natural defenses, as opposed to synthetic or extracted medicines or drugs that work on the body. The body mostly knows what it is doing when it is sick and is simply adapting to the circumstances, doing its best to restore health. Symptoms are a reflection of the body's immune system working to maintain health. However, sometimes the body over reacts or under reacts and needs help to either stimulate or suppress its actions. This is where medicine comes in, either using natural substances that help the body do the work for itself or with synthetic or compounded drugs that do the work for the body. Everything has its place. However, the emphasis in this book is to explore what natural medicine, in particular homeopathy and certain herbal preparations, can do to help in many acute situations, especially when traveling, but also at home. It is important to be informed of all options, and to know the possible choices when dealing with the many challenges and sicknesses that can arise in life.

What is Homeopathy?

Homeopathy is a system of medicine founded by the German physician Samuel Hahnemann, who lived between 1755 and 1843. He wrote six editions of his famous work, The Organon of the Medical Art, which was first published in 1810. Homeopathy spread throughout the world in the nineteenth century and is now practiced on every continent. It is integrated into the health systems of many countries and practiced widely by both physicians, other health professionals and by lay people in the home.

Homeopathy works according to a natural law called the Law of Similars or put another way, **What Can Cause Can Cure.** The premise of homeopathy is that symptoms a substance can cause are the very same symptoms that it can cure, provided it is being given in a specially prepared minimal (micro) dosage. An example would be when cutting an onion. Often one's eyes and nose stream water and if sensitive it can also burn. Therefore, in homeopathy, an onion prepared as a homeopathic remedy is given to treat colds and coughs when the eyes and nose stream and burn. Another example is in looking at the effects of a substance such as Arsenic. It can produce symptoms of diarrhea because of its toxicity, but when prepared as a homeopathic remedy, when only a micro dose of the substance is used, it actually can cure diarrhea. This principle of cure is also called "Like Cures Like".

The principle behind homeopathy is that the substance that most closely matches the symptom picture in a person will work by stimulating the body's own natural intelligence and immune system to cure itself. As the image or impression of the medicine is similar to that of the disease, the remedy is, in a sense, waking the body's own immunity to the disease, encouraging the body to cure itself

Whereas conventional drugs do the work for the body, homeopathic remedies make the body do the work itself. This is the same in all natural medicine. It is working with the body's own healing capacity or to put it another way, with the intelligence of nature itself.

Explain more how it works?

There are common plants in the United States called poison ivy and poison oak that in sensitive people can cause outbreaks of very nasty eruptions, with pustules, itching, redness and swelling, which in some cases can be very serious. In homeopathy, that plant, called *Rhus tox* is excellent to treat actual poison oak and ivy reactions and other 'similar' types of eruptions. it doesn't have to be exactly poison oak. Any similar skin disease may be treated with this homeopathic remedy. "What can cause can cure". It is also known that if you have a mild burn, by putting a mild heat as opposed to cold to the burn, it can alleviate the burning. You do not put intense heat as that would be too much, but just very mild heat. The natural inclination is to put a very cold application to the burn which in intense situations does give immediate relief but soon after that the burning can often get worse. However, when it is slightly better you can put use a somewhat warmer application. This is the application of the homeopathic law, the "Law of Similars".

The founder of homeopathy, Samuel Hahnemann, first explored the homeopathic principle by experimentally taking doses of quinine himself, to see what it would do. He found it produced symptoms similar to malaria, for which quinine had been used for many years. This led him to question whether the fact that it produced symptoms similar to malaria is an indication of its usefulness in its treatment. This led him to further experiment until he could validate that the homeopathic Law of Similars gives us information on the healing power of natural substances. He wasn't the first to consider this concept. Hippocrates, the Greek physician, known as the father of modern medicine also said that one can cure by similars or by opposites. What Hahnemann did was to codify this concept into a system of healing.

What Samuel Hahnemann stumbled on was a method of cure that could activate the body's own immune system, even before much about the immune system was known. But he understood that the body (and mind) has amazing capacities to cure itself. If the body can produce symptoms in the first place, then it can also cure these symptoms. He further understood that symptoms were the body's way of revealing what is wrong. They are signs to pay attention to and at times to find medicines for. The fact remains that if the body could always cure itself, we wouldn't need medicines, but Hahnemann understood that the body can only do so much and at times needs further support.

How is the body's immune system stimulated?

When giving a medicine similar in nature to the symptoms of the disease, there is a slight exaggeration of the existing disease symptoms. This forces the body to respond with the equal and opposite reaction to the stimulus of the remedy. Isaac Newton, the seventeenth century scientist established three laws of motion, the third stating that when a force acts on a body due to another body then an equal and opposite force acts simultaneously on that body. This is basically how a homeopathic remedy works according to the Law of Similars. A visual example is that if you push a swing so far in one direction, it will swing to the opposite direction by a similar force. Similarly, in the body, a homeopathic remedy is encouraging the body to optimize its reaction to a disease by slightly magnifying it. This approach can be applied in psychotherapy when if a person has a strong aversion to something, e.g., animals, one can gradually help by getting the person to look at images of an animal, then perhaps see one in a cage or from a distance and then perhaps to touch one with other people around, all the time gradually introducing 'small micro doses' of the thing they are afraid of. By introducing a small dose of the same thing, the body learns to adjust. This is applying the homeopathic Law of Similars.

What is happening when the body produces symptoms?

It is important to understand that symptoms are only the body's reaction to being sick, whether it is a viral or bacterial infection, or due to some other trauma. A bruise or stiffness is a natural reaction to trauma. The body flooding the area with repair cells and pain is a way to get you to restrict motion. A fever is a natural reaction to an infection and should not be suppressed with aspirin or anti-inflammatory medications as it is serving the body and is an important part of the healing process. The only exception to this is when the fever is getting too high and needs to be controlled. The body has an instinctive natural intelligence, built into the DNA of every cell. It is always seeking an optimal reaction to any disease, to respond as best it can.

Homeopathy is needed when the body is unable or struggles to find the optimal response. If things are getting out of control and the body can't cope, medicine is needed to help the body create the optimal response. It is the symptoms that can tell us which remedy is needed and what needs to be done.

Homeopathy works by optimizing the immune system and the natural intelligence of the body. Conventional medicine helps by doing the work for the body when the body can't do it on its own. To use the metaphor of the body as a building, conventional medicines work like a scaffolding when the building is unstable. Homeopathy works more at the level of the foundations, to strengthen the basic integrity of the building. Both approaches are valid. It just depends what is needed. Conventional medications work best when the body is seriously struggling to cope or its reaction is deficient or too much for the situation. Homeopathy works best when the body can still respond and simply needs stimulation to re-establish balance. In most situations, the body can still respond to stimulation but when seriously compromised it can need support that conventional medicine can offer.

There are many occasions when due to serious acute or chronic disease, the body will not be able to re-establish optimal health any longer. No form of medicine can do everything and if the body has fundamental or structural limitations, then only some improvement is possible. But in nearly all situations, some improvement can be made.

How do symptoms help in finding a homeopathic remedy?

Every time someone gets sick, a unique configuration of symptoms is experienced. Even when people have the same basic disease, whether influenza, a cold or any other condition, it can express a somewhat different picture in various people, therefore requiring a different remedy. Symptoms are expressed in both subjective and objective ways, from the qualities of pain, whether it is burning, stinging or stitching, to the things that make the symptoms better or worse, whether it is movement, pressure, cold or heat, or the time of day a symptom arises. Also the factors that induce a symptom picture, whether it is emotional shock, exposure to cold or heat, or some particular trauma, can inform the choice of a homeopathic (or herbal) remedy. Symptoms are the expression of the disease in the person. They reflect the unique reaction to the disease at any given time.

How do we find the correct remedy for the condition?

Each homeopathic or herbal remedy has its own unique picture based on the symptom picture it has been known to create. In homeopathy this picture is established in an experiment called a proving when a number of healthy people are given small doses of a homeopathic remedy. Instead of animal experimentation with toxic doses of drugs, minute amounts of remedies are given to human volunteers to evaluate their reaction. All the symptoms created during this process are assessed and collated and become the image of the remedy, of what the remedy can cause and can therefore cure. The correct remedy will therefore have a similar symptom image to that of a natural disease state a person is experiencing. Every substance used as a homeopathic remedy has its own picture based on the fact that every substance is unique. Homeopathy finds this unique pattern and matches it to the person's symptoms.

As you become more familiar with the remedies in this book, you will be able to recognize the unique image for each remedy and how the same remedy can be used for many different conditions, irrespective of the diagnosis or name given.

In herbal medicine, the therapeutic action is revealed through many ways, from studying the form, shape and chemical composition of the plant, to its historical use over the centuries and also in experimental settings where the plants' unique qualities are studied and explored.

What are homeopathic remedies made from?

Homeopathic remedies are made from all natural substances, mineral, animal and plant. Most are from plants as there are simply more plants than other substances but all the major minerals and metals, such as potassium, phosphorus and silicea are used in homeopathy, as well as animal based substances, such as snake and spider venom. It is the extraordinary number and the depth of homeopathic remedies that makes it such a fascinating system of healing. In theory, all of nature can be used to heal. Much of modern medicine, even if now in a synthesized form, originated from nature. In homeopathy, the substances used are taken in their whole form most of the time, just as they are found in nature. Conventional medicine, by comparison, often tends to isolate the 'active' ingredient in a substance and to use only that, or mixed with other substances also isolated from their origin. All homeopathic remedies are prepared in specialized pharmacies according to strict criteria, and always in doses that are safe for people. Being prepared in pharmacies means their manufacture is highly regulated, ensuring safety and quality. Homeopathic remedies are always given their Latin name, so wherever you are in the world, you can recognize, ask for or order the name of the remedy.

What is the difference between homeopathic and herbal remedies?

The main difference is in the form of the plant used and the rationale for giving a particular remedy. As mentioned, a homeopathic remedy is given based on the Law of Similars, or Like cures Like - That which can cause symptoms in healthy people will cure similar symptoms in a sick person. That is what makes it homeopathic, not the actual substance used. Secondly, homeopathic remedies are always prepared by homeopathic pharmacies in a form in which they are potentized or energized by a process of dilution and shaking, according to a strict mathematical formula. This potentization process allows the inherent healing power of the remedy to be accessed and at the same time eliminates any possible toxicity in a remedy. That is why in homeopathy, substances such as mercury, gold and even animal venoms can be used. Any potential toxicity has been eliminated by the potentization process.

In herbal medicine, a herb is given in its physical material form, either as a tincture or tea or in a tablet or capsule form. It works primarily by directly affecting the physiology of the body. It may also be working according to the homeopathic law and many herbs do work in a homeopathic way, stimulating the body's immune system and at the same time supporting the physiological function of the body. Many of the herbs mentioned in this book can be given in a homeopathic form as well as a herbal one.

What is meant by the term 'holistic'?

The term holism is used to describe the idea that all things are connected. In terms of the human body, it clarifies the fact that all functions of the mind and body are interconnected and so when one part of the body expresses symptoms, it is still the whole organism that is affected. Separating the functions of the body and mind into different boxes and finding medicines for all the different boxes is not a 'holistic' way of thinking. Also, separating the mind from the body and not recognizing the subtle but profound interconnections is not holistic. The same applies with the relationship we have with our environment and the whole world around us.

Holistic systems of medicine always seek to look at the whole person and to understand that as all parts of the body and mind are connected we need to look at the person as an integrated whole and address the significant causes of any imbalance that leads to disease. Only then are we addressing the roots of illness and not just treating the effect.

How do you treat the causes of any disease?

It depends very much on the particular situation in which a person finds him/herself. In acute diseases, like a cold, a homeopathic or herbal remedy can be given to support the body and help stimulate the body to take care of the problem. The cause is the specific bacteria or virus and the body is reacting to that infection. However, even then, different people will respond in many different ways to the same infection, as their physical and emotional make up are different. For example, if a person has a sore throat after experiencing an emotional upset, the real cause is the emotional upset, not the bacteria that 'caused' the sore throat. Another person may get a similar sore throat but for a different reason. So, in homeopathy one has to individualize each case. The same remedy is not necessarily given to all the people with the same infection. In more chronic and complex conditions, the cause may be much more complicated. It may be a combination of factors, involving family history and genetic predisposition, emotional factors and/or history of other illnesses; or it may be due to some form of physical or psychological shock. In homeopathy, it is important always to put the whole case together, like a jigsaw. It is only when all the pieces of a person's life are put together as a 'whole' can true causes be seen and all the factors that affect a person's health be understood.

So, in homeopathy different remedies can treat the same 'disease'?

Yes. It is commonly said by homeopaths that homeopathy treats the person, not the disease. A disease is a category of symptoms and is given a label, a name. This is useful to know and often the same disease label invites the same drug, irrespective of the differences in the person's expression of the disease. This is part of the conventional model of treatment. It is not bad and in many cases, it works very well in defining appropriate care. However, from a holistic view, especially in more chronic cases, how the whole person is responding and dealing with the disease is taken into consideration. A remedy is found by matching the whole picture including the individual characteristic symptoms of each person. Only by this kind of precision can a homeopathic remedy work. It has to match closely the whole symptom picture. If the wrong remedy is given, then normally nothing happens. The correct remedy, by matching the symptoms of the person to that of the remedy will most accurately stimulate the optimal healing potential in a person. A less precise remedy won't do this.

In more acute illnesses, including epidemics, individual differences are not so apparent. Many people may need the same remedy as they are all under the influence of the same bug, at the same time. One or two remedies only may be needed to treat the epidemic. When the external influence is strong enough, whether an infectious material or some other dramatic circumstance, e.g., experiencing an earthquake, then individual differences are not that important as people are 'sharing' the same experience.

In this book, most situations are more acute and that is why only a limited number of remedies are suggested and also why certain remedies can be used for different conditions. The concept of treating chronic cases is only mentioned to give you an idea of the depth of homeopathy and also to understand the difference between acute and chronic care.

What is the difference between how conventional drugs and natural remedies work?

Conventional drugs work on the body. Essentially they do the work for the body until the body can do the work for itself. Antibiotics kill the bacteria. Drugs often work by suppressing the body's reaction to disease, like an anti-inflammatory drug in arthritis. While that can give great relief, the underlying causes of the condition are not addressed. Conventional drugs work best when the body cannot respond appropriately to disease, whether an acute infection or in more chronic diseases when the body is breaking down and simply needs stability and support. The earlier analogy of the building needing scaffolding fits here.

However, a homeopathic remedy does not work directly on the body but uses the body's own innate intelligence to stimulate the optimal response so the body cures itself. Even in bacterial or viral diseases, a homeopathic remedy works well, but it doesn't directly kill the bacteria, it rather helps the body eliminate them. It makes the terrain of the body less inhabitable for the bacteria or virus.

Are bacteria and viruses the cause of some diseases?

Yes and no. Obviously they are the precipitating cause of many acute infectious diseases, like the common cold and the 'flu. However, it is always seen that only some people catch the bacteria or virus and others don't. More accurately, only some people get sick even if the viruses or bacteria are everywhere. Many bacteria exist normally within the body and it is when some other factors are initiated that they become harmful, e.g., the use of drugs or the introduction of other bacteria. We are not just passive recipients of these bugs. The fundamental quality of our own health is very important. As the scientist Claude Bernard said, and apparently Louis Pasteur (one of the founders of microbiology) also, on his deathbed, "the terrain is everything, the germ nothing." The founder of homeopathy, Samuel Hahnemann, also understood this and focused much of his work in understanding the roots of sickness and why we get sick in the ways we do.

As modern medicine has focused predominantly on killing germs, whether bacteria or viruses, it has paid much less attention to understanding the reasons why bacteria are there in the first place and why some people get sick and others don't. Germs represent an antagonistic part of nature, which needs to be destroyed. However, germs, like any other living thing are merely surviving in the best way they can and are opportunistic. They are attracted to terrain which is already compromised and sick in most cases. Attempting to destroy them with antibiotics has led to the abuse of these medicines and as a result some bacteria have adapted and become immune to antibiotics. This is a huge problem but the issue stems from the idea that we can control nature and that the sole cause of many diseases is due to germs, ignoring the issue of the terrain and why some people get sick and others don't.

Of course, the ability of medicine to kill germs has saved millions of lives, especially since the introduction of antibiotics, which has only been since around 1950. However, we are dealing with the fact that many bacteria are now immune to antibiotics and nature in general is seemingly able to adapt itself to whatever drugs we create. We have to find a different way to deal with many diseases.

How do we affect the terrain of our body?

We need to feed it well and keep it well watered. The terrain of the body is very similar to soil. It needs nourishment but also it has intrinsic limits depending on the bedrock and the environment in which it exists. As so with the body, the genetic disposition plays a big factor in our health, but even here, it is not simple. There is so much we don't know about what initiates disease. For example, the mind-body connection is very important and often very subtle. It is simply not possible to know why we get sick sometimes and many factors are often involved.

A genetic predisposition to an illness doesn't always mean a person will get the disease. We are all different and we respond to life's stresses in different ways. Genetic factors are not so carved in stone when predicting disease, in spite of what some people are saying today. The differences in our DNA are but one factor in determining our health but it is true that coming from a healthy stock of long living people will give you more chances of doing the same.

Keeping the body and mind healthy with good food and good hydration, living in a healthy environment with fresh air, exercise and minimizing stress in life will allow optimal health to be experienced. Also, optimizing a person's immune system with holistic therapies that directly stimulate the body's own defenses and that help balance mind and body, will help prevent all forms of disease. Similar to servicing a car, everybody needs a tune up now and again, to stop the car breaking down or simply to keep the car functioning well. Holistic therapies like homeopathy and herbal medicine can do this. They help balance the whole system so that a person can live a healthy and ideally happy life.

In the context of travel and being prepared for foreign countries and all possible health challenges, some preventative or 'prophylactic' measures need to be taken. This is discussed in Chapter Sixteen, which looks at all forms of prevention. There is only so much one can do though when preparing to travel and of course, the more risks that are taken, the more likely you are to get sick. But traveling does not necessarily mean you have to get sick. Avoiding contaminated food and water, or being bitten by insects that spread diseases and other obvious factors is the best policy. Prevention is better than cure.

Will a healthy constitution help prevent disease?

Yes. The healthier you are in general and the more balanced your life-style, then you are likely to remain healthy. Everybody knows that eating good food is essential to good health, but you wouldn't know that by looking at much of what we eat in modern society or for that matter, the food you find in hospitals. Doctors have historically been taught very little about nutrition and only now is it really being recognized how significant diet can be in preventing many diseases, such as heart disease, diabetes, high blood pressure, high cholesterol, cancer etc. Many of these diseases would be reduced if we changed our diet and also ate less. Many of the chronic ailments we suffer in modern society today is partly due to the amount of bad food eaten. Similarly, the amount of stress that people experience has a profound effect on health. A hundred years ago the stresses of life were often very immediate. Access to a job, food and decent habitation were often a challenge, perhaps compounded by working situations that were physically dangerous and/or environmentally toxic. Disease doesn't happen in a vacuum and often reflects the wider cultural and social situation. That is why the biggest advance in our health in the last 100 years has been clean water and efficient sewage systems. Much more than any medical advances, these social programs transformed our health and eliminated many diseases, which is why when traveling to areas where basic hygiene is a challenge, more care needs to be taken and simple preventative measures understood and adhered to.

Can both conventional drugs and homeopathic remedies be used at the same time?

Yes. In most situations, they can be given together. They will not interfere with one another as they are working on different levels of the body. As mentioned, conventional drugs work directly on the physical body, whereas homeopathic remedies are working to stimulate the body's own healing power. Herbal medicines are different as they also mainly work on the physical body and therefore, it is important to research any possible interference between them and conventional drugs. Any substance, whether natural or synthetic can cause side-effects due to the toxicity of the substance or simply the amount given. Also, some people are more likely to be affected than others, depending on their individual disposition. Homeopathic remedies do not produce side effects. At times the body can produce new symptoms as it is cleaning out the system but that doesn't happen when dealing with acute conditions.

What are the limits to the use of homeopathic and herbal remedies?

It depends on each situation and the capacity of the body to respond to the remedies given. It also depends on taking the right remedy. The wrong remedy will do nothing, so it is not the limits of homeopathy, but the choice of remedy given. The same goes with herbal medicines. However, if a case is serious, one always has to take care and seek appropriate professional medical care and also professional homeopathic or herbal care. One can't do everything on one's own. Also, in possibly serious conditions, such as malaria, typhoid, dysentery, hepatitis etc, it is important to ensure all care is taken and to consult a professional therapist, if at all possible. However, in most acute situations, especially when no other help is available, having a homeopathic first aid kit can be a vital help and give you great confidence in dealing with many situations.

Chapter Two
How To Use Natural Medicine

How to read this book

Each chapter deals with a variety of similar conditions connected by similar causes or which are found in the same region of the body. For each condition, a number of homeopathic and herbal remedies are suggested, along with a brief description of the condition and how it occurs. A detailed list of all the remedies recommended in the book are found in Chapter Seventeen and should be used to complement the information given for each condition. Each remedy may be used for more than one condition and it is useful to have an understanding of the main characteristics of each remedy. The more familiar you are with the qualities of each remedy, the more easily you will recognize them in yourself and friends when they are needed.

The information presented is not meant to take the place of conventional medical care or the advice of your physician. However, it does offer an alternative to conventional care if that care is not working or is not available. Homeopathic and herbal remedies can also be used in conjunction with other alternative and conventional medicines. For each condition, a number of homeopathic remedies are suggested, followed by other natural approaches that can be used at the same time. It is not always easy to find the correct homeopathic remedy for a condition as there are often different possibilities. This book attempts to simplify that process for the reader and make the choice of remedy that much easier. If it seems difficult to choose the correct remedy, the reader has to pick one remedy or put more than one remedy together by mixing them in water and taking or giving it in a liquid form. Directions of how to give the remedy(ies) will follow.

Homeopathic remedies are not only given according to a disease diagnosis but to a unique group of symptoms, which can be potentially seen in many different disease states. It is important to recognize the key qualities in each medicine and identify those key features when they appear in a particular condition. For example, the remedy *Arsenicum album* is useful in both diarrhea and also various fevers, but one has to see some qualities of burning pains, restlessness, anxiety and chilliness to justify the remedy, whatever the condition and name of the disease. However, not all the symptoms of a remedy have to be there to give that remedy. A select few is enough but the symptoms have to be the most characteristic ones that the person is experiencing and that are found in the remedy.

All homeopathic remedies are given their Latin name. This is consistent throughout the world. Homeopathic remedies can be found in many countries, including all of Europe, the United States, Central and South America, Canada, Australasia, India, Pakistan, Bangladesh, Sri Lanka and Russia. In most countries, the remedies will be made according to strict criteria and are trustworthy. If you are in any doubt, please consult a homeopathic consultant and ask them. Homeopathic remedies are freely available to buy in most countries, either from pharmacies or natural food stores (if they exist). Otherwise, you can purchase them through homeopathic doctors.

See Chapter Eighteen, Resources and References

How to take homeopathic remedies

In general, you can give/take one or two globules/tablets, put it/them into your mouth and let dissolve. It doesn't matter though if you chew it. Do not take anything else at the same time as you take the remedy, including water, tea or coffee. Take the remedy dry. Ensure your mouth is clean and has nothing else in it. Only handle it if your hands are clean. Otherwise, use the lid of the bottle. Do not touch a remedy if it is for somebody else.

If a remedy is to be repeated frequently (more than twice a day), it is best to dissolve one or more globules/tablets into two to four ounces of water and take one teaspoon according to the frequency indicated, which depends on the severity of the symptoms. Even a remedy to be taken three to four times a day can be done this way and, each day, make a new batch with fresh water and another globule/tablet. The water should be stirred or shaken well each time before taking a teaspoon of the liquid. It makes no difference in terms of strength if the remedy is taken dry or in liquid form. If a tablet is dissolved into a small amount of water, the imprint of the remedy is infused into the water and it will have the same effect as taking a tablet on the tongue. What is important is the potency/strength of the remedy and how often it is repeated.

In more extreme situations, e.g., a high fever or intense pain, a remedy can be taken every one to five minutes, or every fifteen minutes to every hour, depending on the situation. You can't really take too much of a remedy. Your body will take what it needs and when symptoms subside then you can simply stop or reduce the remedy. In more chronic situations, like an old strain or injury, then taking one tablet daily for one week will be enough. It will need some time to see major improvement. On average, you will be taking or giving a remedy one to three times a day.

The same applies to the potency (strength) of the remedy. Each homeopathic remedy is given a number after its name. This relates to the potency of the remedy and the strengths are often as follows - 6c, 30c, 200c, 1m and 10m. The higher numbers relate to a higher or stronger potency and are usually used in more serious conditions. However, for practical purposes, only 30c and 200c are recommended here as these are potencies that come with kits and that are more widely available. They are also strong enough for most situations.

Some remedies may be mentioned that are not included in the kits used with this book. These remedies would have to be purchased separately, either locally or online. A list of all the remedies mentioned in the book and in the kits available are on the following website: **www.thenaturalmedicineguide.com**. If you think that one of the remedies listed could be needed, due to particular travel plans or prior experience, then it is good to get this remedy in advance.

Alternatively, you may want to consider some herbal medicines to complement the homeopathic remedy given. The dosages will also depend on the severity of the condition and instructions should be followed for each condition, which are found on the label of all herbal preparations. Generally, homeopathic and herbal preparations can be given in conjunction with any conventional medicines being taken but especially with herbal preparations it is important to pay attention to any potential interactions between the two. If you have any questions, do consult your prescribing doctor and read labels of all preparations.

How to take herbal remedies

Herbal remedies should generally be taken according to instructions that come with them if they are bought in a packaged form. However, given that herbs are physical substances with possible side-effects, it is important to note any effects and to stop if symptoms are getting worse or new conditions develop. It is also important to follow any recommended information for children and pregnant women. If herbs are taken in a loose form, being made up on the spot or in places where it is not possible to evaluate the dosage, caution should be taken and it is good to start with a small amount and note the effect and gradually build up if it seems fine to do so. It is also worth asking people who have experience with local herbs.

How to keep remedies safe

Homeopathic remedies will stay effective for an indefinite amount of time if they are looked after, irrespective of any expiry date on the label, which is done to comply to the law. They should be kept in a water proof container and be kept as dry as possible. Sometimes in the tropics they can get moist but try and keep them dry. Do not expose remedies to direct sunlight or very strong smells, like eucalyptus, camphor etc. Avoid too intense heat. If pills escape and fall to the table or floor, do not put them back in the bottle. Prolonged exposure to X- rays may antidote the remedies. However, it is now unavoidable if one travels by air as all baggage is X-rayed. It seems that remedies work well after exposure to X-rays when traveling, but it is worth paying attention if much travel is done over a number of years as their strength may be eroded over time.

Evaluating the action of homeopathic remedies

Homeopathic remedies will generally work according to the needs of the body. In intense situations in which there is a high fever, acute pain or some other very acute situation, the remedy will work in between one and fifteen minutes. In less severe situations, some change will be seen in one to four hours. For example, in a sprained ankle without much pain, relief will be seen in twelve hours to two days. A simple case of diarrhea may take one day to get better. A more intense case may take longer but some improvement in most cases will be seen in the first day. One does have to have some patience though. Do not panic just because you have diarrhea and take every over-the-counter medicine possible. Give the body a chance. One has to assess the needs of the situation to the action of the remedy.

In intense situations, when a remedy works, the first reaction is often that the person falls asleep. This is a good sign. Once there is a clear sign of the remedy working, then the remedy can be stopped or given less frequently. Use your judgment. If pain disappears totally, stop the remedy. If symptoms begin to return, begin the remedy again, repeating at suitable intervals. There is some flexibility here. If a remedy is working, do not change it. Continue it less frequently until it has completed its action. Also, consider a higher potency of the same remedy if it initially worked well and then seems to stop working.

Sometimes the remedy is only partially effective as it is not the exact one needed, but it will still work somewhat and perhaps another remedy will follow to finish things off. Pay attention to how well a remedy works and always keep other possible remedies in mind. Look at the other remedies listed for the same condition.

One of the first signs of improvement is an increase in energy and well being, even if the symptoms persist. This is good. In time the

symptoms will get better. If symptoms seem to get a little worse immediately after taking a remedy, it is usually a sign that the body is being
activated through the remedy and relief should soon set in. The rule
generally is that the more intense the situation, the quicker the remedy
will work. It may take only seconds to see relief or it may take a number
of hours and even days in situations that are more long term.

Trust the remedy. If it is correct it will work and it will work quickly
if need be.

Terminology

- **SD** Single dose (usually taken once daily).
- **Allopathy** Term used in homeopathy to describe conventional
  medicine
- **Acute condition** A self limiting condition that may often
  require support but will normally resolve by itself in time.
- **Chronic condition** A longer standing condition that normally
  will not resolve by itself, requiring homeopathic constitutional
  care by a professional, or some other form of therapy.
- **Constitution** Relates to the basic physical and psychological
  characteristics of a person.
- **Nosode** A homeopathic remedy made from diseased material,
  e.g., discharge from bacterial infections.
- **6x, 12x, 6c, 30c and 200c, 1m, 10m** This relates to the
  strength of the homeopathic medicine. Potencies with an **x**
  after have been mixed in a ratio of 1/10 (that is one drop of the
  substance mixed with 10 drops of water). Those with a **c** after
  have been mixed in the ration of 1/100. Take each remedy as
  indicated but if a 200c is indicated and you only have a 30c,
  then take that instead. In this book, only **c** potencies are being
  recommended, mostly 30c and at times 200c, but if you can
  only get **x** potencies somewhere, that will work fine.

Chapter Three
Being Prepared

It is useful to research the types of health challenges one can face in the countries being visited. This way, you can be forewarned and take all necessary precautions. This is not just for medical reasons but also to understand the culture you may be visiting and the various norms of that culture, including food habits.

Many of the conditions found in this book are only found in certain areas of the world. Knowing the likelihood of getting any of these diseases can help you in your preparation and to know what preventative measures to take. This is discussed more in Chapter Sixteen: Prevention. Also, if you have particular nutritional needs, knowing what foods may be available may also be important. Eating local food is often one of the interesting parts of travel, but is also one of the riskiest activities in terms of getting sick.

If you are embarking on more arduous journeys requiring special preparation, then doing the necessary research ahead of time is invaluable. See Chapter Seventeen: Resources and References for some recommendations of research materials.

Avoiding getting sick is the best strategy when traveling or for that matter, at any time. Most diseases travelers get are passed on through contaminated food and water. By far the most common conditions experienced are some form of diarrhea due to bad food, more so than water. Therefore being prudent in this area is crucial for well being.

Other forms of prevention can involve taking natural medicines, supplements and also conventional medicines. One of the most common forms of conventional prevention used is vaccinations or immunizations. Discussion of vaccinations with their risks and benefits and natural options are given in Chapter Sixteen: Prevention.

Minimize infections

It is impossible to avoid coming across a multitude of infectious agents when traveling, especially in more challenging places. Part of this is due to our contact with unfamiliar bugs we have little immunity to, partly the circumstances we find ourselves in, especially eating out and often the hygiene challenges we may come across. However, the body is generally a resilient thing and after a while, some natural immunity is developed. But it is not uncommon when traveling to get at least one dose of diarrhea or a cold of some sort.

However, take all precautions to prevent infection. Wash your hands a lot, especially before and after eating. Take your own liquid soap with you. Also use anti-bacterial wipes or gels to prevent infections. This is especially useful when water is not available or if you have to use water and your hand to clean yourself after going to the bathroom. This is a very common practice in much of the world and is very hygienic as long as you can wash your hands afterwards. Don't walk barefoot apart from on beaches. You can catch various little creatures and also injure your feet, which is often a source of infection in tropical areas.

Food and Water

It is imperative to avoid drinking bad water or contaminated food. They account for a majority of diseases travelers get on the road, including diarrhea, dysentery, cholera, typhoid, hepatitis A etc. Bad food is sometimes harder to avoid now than bad water, so particular attention should be given to the food eaten. Drink bottled water or boil your water. Also take water sterilization methods with you. Iodine or chlorine is best.

Even cleaning your teeth in tap water should be avoided unless you know the water is OK. In restaurants plates and cutlery can still be wet and should be wiped clean. Carry a clean small towel or wipes with you.

Common sense is important. Always check out the places to eat and where you get your water from. Research the good bottled water companies. They are not all the same. Also, sometimes there are scams to refill empty water bottles so check the lid is sealed and the water tastes OK. Some water tastes like gasoline due to the process of filtering and sterilizing. Do not drink it. Luckily, this happens less now than it used to. Do not put your lips to any bottle that somebody else has drunk from. Avoid ice and ice cream as this is very risky. Commercial soft drinks are generally OK and sodas can be useful to help a mild upset stomach. Some local brands may not be that good and can at times have nasty chemicals in so it is best to ask around what people drink. However, it is best not to drink too many sodas and to hydrate with water and other natural liquids. Fresh coconut water is excellent for hydration and general health.

Badly prepared food is the major form of catching bacteria, viruses and parasites. It is important to check out as much as possible the quality of a place before eating. The following are a few hints

- Eat where locals eat, (within the boundaries of normal hygiene). Does the place seem busy and active.
- A fancy restaurant does not necessarily indicate a clean kitchen but avoid 'dumps'.
- Avoid any food that tastes 'bad'. (I know that sounds obvious but at times we continue to eat something we shouldn't. Meat and fish particularly need close attention).
- Avoid uncooked food, including salads (unless you can be sure it has been cleaned thoroughly). Especially avoid lettuce. Peel all raw vegetables and fruit. Avoid mayonnaise as it may carry salmonella. Fresh yoghurt is OK but even then, be careful.
- Avoid raw or undercooked meat or fish in any form. It is best to stick to a more vegetarian diet in many countries. Meat is often not kept in a hygienic way and is a vector for some very unpleasant bugs. Fish can also be a problem, especially shell fish.

If eating fish, ensure it is cooked well and generally avoid shell fish. Avoid all fish caught in contaminated waters, for example, during red tides (when many fish die for various reasons and pollute the sea). Always check with locals what fish are good to eat. All milk should be boiled before drinking. Even boiled milk left to cool can quickly become infected. Minimize consumption of dairy food and eggs.

- Avoid food that has been re-cooked or re-heated, including rice. Fried rice is very suspect as often it is slightly reheated from a previous meal. If food is meant to be hot, make sure it is hot when you eat it.
- Eat what the locals are eating. Do not ask for foods that they are not that familiar with.
- Don't pick your own berries or other wild food – including mushrooms - unless you are sure you know what it is. It may look like a plant back home but it could be poisonous.

Discussions and theories about basic nutrition are seemingly more complex than religion. Endless theories about diet are continually being debated with 'new' diets constantly emerging, whether for weight loss or optimal nutrition. Modern agricultural methods are producing vegetables with less of the essential vitamins and minerals we need and it is debatable if many people, even in developed economies, are getting enough essential nutrition. Therefore a good quality vitamin and mineral supplement, (which are food based as opposed to synthetically based) is recommended as part of one's daily nutrition. However, when traveling it is not crucial to take supplements with you especially if traveling for only short periods. There is fresh food easily available in most developing countries and the diet may be simple but fairly healthy.

If you eat meat, then ideally you should know where it comes from and what the animal is being fed. That means eating locally produced organic meat. The industrial meat industry, especially in the United States, is producing meat that is often full of hormones and antibiotics. They are often kept in horrendous conditions, which must affect the quality of meat, let alone the ethical considerations, making eating such meat a health risk. Eating organic meat is much more important than eating organic fruit and vegetables. However, especially in the United States, the introduction of genetically modified (GM) foods into the food supply makes eating organic and local produce more important. In spite of all the ideas floating around about diets and the importance of nutrition, it is fair to say that if one sticks to eating as many vegetables as possible and a reasonable amount of fruit (in tropical climes, fruit becomes a greater proportion in ones diet), eating whole grains mainly (brown rice, quinoa, oats), pulses (lentils, all sorts of beans) and small amounts of fish and meat if you choose to, is a good diet. Avoid too much dairy and use olive oil for most cooking. Coconut and Sesame oil are also good. Avoid all margarines and also canola oil which are too processed. Palm oil is fairly ubiquitous in Africa and parts of South America, but this should be used sparingly. Ghee (clarified butter) is common in India and is generally fine. Avoid too much sugar, although this is easier said than done in many countries. However, at home, it is not so hard. Wean yourself off sugar in your coffee and tea if you can. There is a growing epidemic of diabetes in both developed and developing countries. Diet is a major factor.

Hydration

It is very important when visiting warm humid countries to stay hydrated. Drinking enough is crucial for well-being and to avoid dehydration. This is especially the case when exerting oneself and sweating a lot. So make sure you drink enough water. Take your own water bottle with you, ideally made from stainless steel. Plastic bottles deteriorate and the hard plastic bottles leach chemicals over time and when exposed to the sun. If you do become dehydrated, for whatever reason, drink small amounts to begin with. Do not drink too much at first. However, before any exertion, walking in the heat etc., take in as much water as you can. Prevention again is the best option. Once you have drunk a lot before exertion, resist taking in more water until you really have to. If you do drink more water, most of it is simply sweated away. Drink only when you really need to if you are dealing with a limited water supply. Pay attention to the symptoms of dehydration - dark, odorous urine, difficult respiration, stiffness of joints, excessive tiredness. Carry rehydration tablets with you if think there is any chance of becoming dehydrated.

Rehydration can help with many conditions. Obviously treating a disease like cholera requires instant rehydration, but even for situations like jetlag, altitude sickness and tiredness from being in a hot, tropical situation can benefit from using rehydration mixtures. Any diarrhea that continues more than 24 hours or is particularly strong is a good reason to use them. However, with any diarrhea, simply drink more water and other fluids. Do not drink milk. If you don't have rehydration mixtures, use the following equation: one teaspoon of salt with eight teaspoons of sugar and one liter of clean water. You don't want it too salty. If making a smaller amount, use a pinch of salt to one to three tsp. of sugar. Honey, brown sugar, molasses etc., are fine to use instead of white sugar. You can also add a pinch of salt to a soft drink instead. It may taste bad, but it will work. Generally avoid hot drinks to rehydrate, but lukewarm drinks are OK, including various teas and even weak coffee. Do not drink alcohol to attempt to rehydrate.

If you feel dizzy or have a headache with diarrhea you may be dehydrated and you have to drink more. Oral rehydration mixtures (ORS) can be taken if you are a diabetic but an acute diarrhea may upset sugar levels.

Adjusting to a very warm climate can be one of the most challenging things for those unused to such climates. The heat can be enervating and some constitutions are very challenged by such situations. This is why it is crucial to maintain your water intake. Drink a lot.

Ensure the water is clean. If offered a glass of water that has not been treated, refuse unless you are sure it is OK. Take a cup of tea instead. Even if that water is not totally boiled, hot water still kills many bugs. Boil your water before drinking. Boil for about two minutes. If at higher altitudes, boil the water longer. For example at 5,000 ft, boil it for at least five minutes. Once the water is boiled, do not put it into an untreated or used plastic bottle. Do sterilize any water bottles you are using by pouring boiling water into them.

If it is not possible to boil the water and no other treated water is available, get a plastic bottle, put some water in it, and leave it in the sun for about five hours. In that time, many of the bugs would be killed. If the water is still murky one can filter it through a sock if the material is woven tight enough. This is just in emergencies. There are various forms of filtration equipment that are effective in cleaning water of most bugs. However, they are often awkward to use and carry and are not always that effective. They are more useful as part of using chemical sterilization or when you will be in one place for quite a while, instead of moving around a lot. However, some portable filter bags are useful to have if you are in the 'bush' and the water is particularly murky. Chemical sterilization is useful to have if you are doing any kind of traveling in areas where you cannot find access to good bottled water. It is worth finding out ahead of time what the situation is in the places you may be going to. The two main forms of sterilization are using chlorine and iodine. Both work. Chlorine tastes worse. They may not kill cysts that can cause dysentery and giardiasis unless the dose is high enough (five to ten drops per liter or one tablet per liter). However, do check this information when buying chlorine or iodine equipment.

If you are sweating a lot, you should ensure that you are getting enough salt. Simply use more salt on your food. Normally your body will crave more salt but pay attention to this and use a little more. A refreshing drink to take is carbonated or still water, with fresh limes or lemons squeezed in and a pinch of salt.

Travel

The actual process of travel takes its toll, from stiffness and sleeplessness to travel sickness and the need to be aware of deep vein thrombosis (DVT). Any long trip should involve being able to stand, stretch and loosen up the body. Especially stretch the legs by pointing the feet forward and then flexing the feet back. A DVT comes when due to blood collecting in the lower limbs, a clot forms which then travels up the body into various organs, which can kill. So, especially when traveling by air, make sure you get up frequently, stretch and walk about. Also to avoid DVT, stay well hydrated and avoid wearing tight socks. Jet lag is another common experience, which cannot really be avoided but can be minimized by staying hydrated, minimizing alcohol and by trying to sleep. Taking a natural or conventional sleeping aid may be useful in helping to get some sleep. See Chapter Four: Jet lag section for remedy choices for both prevention and treatment.

If you are feeling sick when traveling or know you get travel sickness or have been sick and then have to travel, take precautions before your journey. Consider taking conventional medications to prevent nausea and sickness. Take some plastic bags with you just in case!
See Chapter Four: Accidents, Injuries and Trauma, Travel Sickness section.

Heat

One of the big adjustments to tropical travel is dealing with the heat, especially humid heat. Many parts of the world, including Latin and South America, Africa and Asia have very hot climates and for those from northern climes, it can be overwhelming. Some people deal with heat much better than others. Overexposure to the sun and heat in general should be avoided. Dehydration, as discussed, is a major risk of travel and you need to be aware of this at all times especially when exerting yourself in hot climates. Give yourself some time to adjust to a new climate on arrival. Don't rush out on the first day and overdo it. There can be a tendency to want to have air conditioning wherever you stay, but it is best to resist this. Going from one extreme to another is not healthy and you do not adjust to the heat so easily. There are times when it can be a refuge, especially if the nights are extremely hot but do not overdo the A/C option. Wearing a hat can be invaluable when out in the sun and if you dampen it, it can help you stay cool. Make sure you take one with you. Balding heads are particularly susceptible to sunburn and it doesn't take long to get burnt.

Equipment and supplies

Being prepared before travel saves a lot of time. If you are traveling and suddenly need something, it often becomes a hassle to find it. This is both for basic supplies as well as medical equipment. While this book is focusing on natural medicine for both travel and home, having a good basic medical kit with you is very helpful.

Also, ensure you take the right clothing. Shoes especially should be worn in before leaving, particularly if trekking. Take a good pair of sandals and/or flip flops, which are useful to wear in showers and other 'dubious' places. However, don't feel you have to spend a fortune on all sorts of travel gear, even if trekking. There can be a compulsion to be over prepared and you end up carrying way too much stuff. Often you can figure out what you need when you arrive, unless you really know certain things are not going to be available there.

In terms of general supplies you should always include the following: (This is mainly a list that also pertains to health. There are many other individual items you may need and have to be prepared to have).

- 2 torches (flashlights), one hand held and the other attached to the head. You should take AA or AAA batteries or take a wind up flashlight which doesn't use batteries.
- Enough batteries to fit your devices. They are not always easy to find or of good quality when traveling.
- Alarm clock or cellular phone. Ensure the phone is unlocked so you can get a local SIM card if traveling for any length of time.
- Pens - enough for yourself and to give away. Ball point pens make excellent gifts for children.
- Electronic reader - Ipad, Kindle, Nook etc. Given the ever increasing restrictions on weight allowance when flying, this can be especially useful and also, as long as you have access to wireless phone lines, you can get downloads. It is also good for guidebooks if you don't want to lug one with you as well as medical information and this book.
- Stainless steel water container (minimum of 1 liter).
- Map of the area traveling in. Often they are better quality in your own country than where you are visiting.
- A small travel towel that dries quickly. I always travel with an Indian wrap around 'sarong', which serves as a towel and also for general wear whenever you need to put something on.
- A wash cloth. Very useful when having a bucket wash and using a limited amount of water.
- A pocket knife (with scissors). Tweezers if not part of the knife.

- Sunscreen if you will need it but only use it when necessary. People tend to lavish it on their bodies because of fear of skin cancer. However, unless you are at high risk or have moles that may turn cancerous, it is best to use sunscreen only until you have turned brown and then decrease its use. Most sunscreens are fairly toxic. There is also some evidence that using sun glasses all the time may lessen your skin's ability to adapt to the sun, so the skin gets more easily burnt. This is due to the lack of melanin being released to the skin as the sunglasses give the impression to the brain that you are not in the sun. Fairer people and those whose skin is more at risk should always be careful in the sun.
- Sunglasses, if you are going to be in very bright sunlight for prolonged periods of time. Increased cataracts are a direct result of too much light exposure, e.g., hiking in high altitudes and in the snow. However, as mentioned, they do not need to be used for general sunlight unless you are particularly sensitive to sunlight. Ensure you get good quality glasses.
- Spare reading glasses.

Medical supplies

- Insect repellent: (See Chapter Sixteen: Prevention, Malaria). A DEET based repellent (30-50%) is important in malaria infested areas. Clothes, especially socks, can also be soaked in repellant for extra protection. A roll-on stick or spray is most efficient. I find the sprays more messy. Natural insect repellants such as citronella and eucalyptus mixed together in an alcohol based spray can be used as a daily repellent and should be taken as well.
- Mosquito coils (although these are commonly found in most mosquito infested places).
- Antiseptic wipes.
- Band-aids of various sizes and some non stick dressings and tape. Steristrips. Blister aids if walking a lot (moleskin, and special tape for blisters).

- Oral rehydration (ORS) if you are going to be in remote and/or very hot places.
- Hypodermic syringes, just in case you need injections and you don't want to be using old syringes.

You may choose to take some conventional medications with you in case of emergency. This can include antibiotics to treat local skin infections, respiratory conditions and the variety of digestive issues commonly experienced. It may also include antihistamines and some painkillers. You should consult your doctor before traveling as to what is possible and appropriate. If going to tropical areas, it may be better to consult a tropical specialist. However, ideally most conditions can be treated with natural medicines and antibiotics etc., can be saved for emergencies only. Don't feel the need to take strong antibiotics at the beginning of any condition. Also, be careful buying medications abroad. In developing countries, many can be fake or dangerous, so only buy from a reputable source.

The Natural Medicine Guide For Travel And Home

Chapter Four
Accidents, Injuries, Trauma

It is important to pay attention to any injury and treat it accordingly. Homeopathic remedies have an affinity for various types of injuries, whether a blow or a cut and also for certain types of tissues e.g., ligaments and muscles, and areas of the body. It is useful to know which remedies address the different tissues of the body and the nature of injuries they cover. It is always important to pay close attention to any injury in case of shock or damage to internal parts of the body and bleeding. What may seem superficial may in fact be a more serious injury. More than one remedy may be needed to affect a cure. Always treat the physical and or mental shock first before going to other remedies. Most likely this will be *Arnica* in physical shock and *Aconite* in mental shock. Please look at the various subsections below for more information.

Accidents and Injury

This is a catch all phrase to cover the variety of situations which need to be treated due to a trauma to the body, including injuries to bones, ligaments, tendons and muscles. It is amazing how effective homeopathic remedies can be in treating all forms of trauma, including sporting injuries and also just the physical stress from over exertion. Prevention is better than cure and taking necessary precautions before strenuous exercise is important. Try not to overdo things at the beginning of any physical exertion. Be prepared, drink and eat enough and don't put your body through too much stress. It can take days to recover and limit your enjoyment and ability to enjoy your experience. Take homeopathic *Arnica* to help prevent stiffness and exhaustion from too much exertion. If you know you are going to over-exert yourself, e.g., competing in a long run or cycle ride, take *Arnica*, one tablet a day for up to three days before the event and three times a day during the event.

If you get wet through from walking through rivers, lakes or due to any other factors, have another set of clothes to change into. Don't stay too long in wet clothes. Be prepared. If you get really chilled, get warm as soon as possible. If you get seriously chilled and can't get warm, take homeopathic *Aconite* (see below).

Even when an injury is more serious and muscles, tendons, ligaments or bones are damaged, homeopathic remedies can facilitate their healing and speed recovery. Different types of injuries are given their own subsection below, but as you will see, many of the same remedies are indicated for different injuries. It is worth reading the whole section to get a good idea of the images for each remedy and the types of injuries covered.

● HOMEOPATHIC CARE

In the beginning of any injury, *Arnica* is the first remedy to give. It is the best remedy for any physical shock or blow, especially with bruising. If you are trekking, it is useful to take it during the first day of hiking when it is easy to overdo it. Take one tablet two to three times that day. Often people walk much further than they should and suffer the consequences. *Arnica* will help here. If you feel any soreness and bruised feeling with any injury, especially to soft tissues, take *Arnica* first. It is also the first remedy for any concussion. Often you can think things are OK and you may say everything is fine when it is not. If you are around any injury in which a person says they are fine, give *Arnica* and wait and observe. If, after an injury there is more emotional shock, with residual fright, *Aconite* is the first remedy to give, one tablet hourly for four hours, before considering other remedies for the physical injury.

If bruising and swelling does not go away after a few days or only is partly helped, *Ledum* should be given, especially in cases of a black eye with residual swelling or bruised feeling, or in injuries to soft tissue, joints and muscles. It is the first remedy to give for punctured wounds and swelling, whether a bite from an insect or a penetrating wound like a nail. It helps prevent tetanus. It is also good for sprains to joints, with puffy swelling and a cold feeling of the injured part. In penetrating punctured wounds, if the pains are extreme and shooting from the injured part, then *Hypericum* should be given. *Hypericum* is excellent for injuries to nerve rich areas where the pains are shooting, sharp and very intense, e.g., injuries to fingers and lacerations to nerve rich areas as well as injuries to the spine, especially the coccyx and the back of the head (occipital).

When the injury is more to the muscles, ligaments, tendons and joints, then *Rhus tox* and *Ruta grav* are remedies to consider. If you have any kind of joint or muscle sprain, whether a hamstring, or injury to the elbow, shoulder, ankle or knee, then these two remedies are important. There can often be a sore, bruised, stiffness in the injured part, which is better through moving it for a while, but then becomes worse from overuse. There can be swelling in the injured area but often the pain improves with warmth. *Ruta grav* is the first remedy for tennis elbow and simple eyestrain from too much reading and is indicated in injuries to smaller joints, like wrists and ankles. *Rhus tox* is indicated for larger joints and muscles, e.g., shoulder joints and hamstrings.

Bryonia is useful for injuries involving joints and bones and often is used in alternation with *Rhus tox*. In *Bryonia*, initially you do not want to move the injured part at all. Everything is made worse from any motion and you want to keep it totally still. Later, as stiffness becomes stronger, then movement may make it feel better, indicating *Rhus tox*. *Bryonia* can be given when there is a broken bone when any movement is unbearable.

Symphytum is excellent for broken bones. Commonly known as knit bone, it helps unite bones once they have been set. It is good for fractures of the cheek bone.

Calendula is a remedy applied locally in a tincture and/or cream as well as an internal remedy. It is useful for any wounds, especially cuts, lacerations and punctured wounds. It is a great healing agent and antiseptic. Some tincture should be put into warm water and the injured area cleaned thoroughly. Internally it is given in a tablet form when lacerations are very painful.

NOTE Often more than one remedy can be needed and often it begins with *Arnica* and then moves to another remedy, depending on the nature of the symptoms and the exact tissues most affected.

✿ HERBAL CARE

Calendula cream and comfrey cream are used for open wounds. If wounds are deep though, a tincture of calendula should be used instead. Lavender, eucalyptus and tea tree oils also can be used.

Altitude Sickness

Altitude sickness happens when a person ascends to a high altitude too quickly. The body struggles to adapt to this change of altitude, not being able to get enough oxygen from the air. The symptoms can be fairly mild to life threatening, depending on the altitude, the rapidity of the ascent and the sensitivity of each person. Symptoms include dizziness, nausea, fatigue, confusion, weakness, headache, breathlessness and palpitations. Symptoms may be acute and quite sudden or gradually develop. This can be a life threatening condition and should not be neglected. All appropriate medical care should be given.

● GENERAL CARE

Do not ascend more than 2,000 feet (600 meters) in one day where you intend to stay overnight. If symptoms are intense, then slowly descend to a lower level of altitude. Do not overexert yourself. Drink a lot of water. You have to avoid any dehydration.

● HOMEOPATHIC CARE

The first remedy to consider is homeopathic *Coca*. Take one tablet every thirty minutes until relief. If that doesn't work or you don't have that remedy, take *Arnica* every thirty minutes. (As *Coca* is made from the plant that cocaine is derived from, it is not so easily available over the counter in pharmacies, even though the homeopathic dosage is just a highly diluted form of the plant).

✎ HERBAL CARE

Chewing coca leaves may have the same effect as the homeopathic *Coca*. (Please check for legality in regards to taking coca leaves. For example, taking coca leaves in Peru may be fine, but it is not OK to take them across the border to Brazil). Taking coca tea works best.

Bites and Stings

The treatment of bites partly depends on what has bitten you. Most nasty bites are from creatures that emit poisons, the most serious being jelly fish, spiders and snakes. However, various insect bites can also be quite serious. Secondary infection of bites, especially in tropical areas is an important consideration and care needs to be taken. Most bites are not serious however. The localized area often becomes swollen and can be painful. This is the natural reaction of the body. In itself, it is not a cause for concern, although any bite needs to be appropriately cleaned to prevent infection. One particular type of bite needs to be discussed is a dog bite, especially in countries where rabies exists. If there is any doubt, you must see a physician and have it checked out. One other important factor is the possible diseases that the bites can spread. This is especially the case for diseases such as malaria, yellow fever, dengue fever, Lyme disease, etc. See each of these conditions for more information.

For prevention of bites and stings, see Chapter Sixteen: Prevention, Malaria section. Always wear shoes when in tropical areas, apart from the beach. This way you can avoid picking up infections and also little insects called jiggers that burrow under the skin, causing pain and infection. If you do get them, they need to be removed with a sterilized needle. Hookworms are also avoided this way. See Chapter Twelve: Skin Conditions, for other affections such as fleas, bedbugs and lice. Also, see Chapter Fourteen: Other Tropical and Infectious Diseases, Leishmaniasis which is caused by the bites of sand flies. For tick bites see Chapter Fifteen: Tick Bite Diseases. Leeches are another attraction of tramping through tropical forests. Having blood filled shoes and socks while walking for miles is one of those unique experiences of travel as is also finding a bloated leech on part of your body! Avoiding leeches is not easy. Wearing boots doesn't work often as they get through the lace holes. Wearing shorts and sneakers can be better as you are more likely to see them as they climb on your shoe or up your leg!

● GENERAL CARE

Ensure any bite or sting is clean. Initially the bite (or wound) should be cleaned well with warm water and soap, washing the wound for at least five minutes. In the case of a bite from a dog the wound should then be washed in alcohol (isopropyl alcohol or even vodka) to further clean the wound. See Chapter Fourteen: Other Tropical and Infectious Conditions, Rabies. *Calendula* tincture and/or *Echinacea* tincture should also be used. If any insect bite is stinging and burning, use *Urtica urens* tincture or cream or any other natural relief for stings. You can also use tea tree or lavender. There are bites from flies that can be very painful and need both local and internal treatment. Also some flies called botflies or tumbu flies can lay larvae that burrow under the skin and can be very painful. If you come back from tropical parts and seem to have something that looks like a cyst under the skin, get it checked out. If still in the tropics try and bring the larvae to the surface by putting paraffin on the infected part or again try using essential oils like tea tree. For leeches, try and remove them by either scraping them off the skin, putting tea tree on them or salt. Once removed, use some tea tree or calendula solution to clean the wound. If you are walking barefoot in water and stand on a sea urchin, put the skin of a papaya on the wound and it will help extract the spine of the fish. Otherwise, getting it out can be difficult and painful.

The first remedies to consider for the effects of simple bites are *Apis* and *Ledum*. *Ledum* is the main remedy for punctured wounds of all sorts, including that of animal bites. The local area may get puffy and swollen, which although may be red in color, may even feel cold. It is best to start with this remedy if no other remedy stands out. *Apis* can either follow *Ledum* or be given first if the bitten area is red, swollen and hard, and has stinging or burning pain. *Apis* will often be needed for the stings of poisonous animals, such as wasps and bees and also if there is any kind of systemic allergic reaction to any bites. In case of a systemic reaction to a bee sting, medical intervention may be necessary. The worst case scenario is a person who goes into anaphylactic shock. This needs immediate medical intervention but *Apis* can be given every one minute while getting attention.

Hypericum can often follow *Ledum*, especially when the bite or sting is very painful and pains shoot along the nerve endings from the area of the bite. *Lachesis* can be needed when the bite looks as though it is becoming infected, turning a bluish/purple or black color or becoming abscessed. You may feel intense burning or stitching pain in the wound. This is often due to venomous bites, especially of snakes and spiders. *Crotalus horridus* (a remedy made from the venom of a rattlesnake) can also be considered when the local swelling becomes blue/black and the blood from the wound is also black. The snake remedies are considered more when there are serious toxic effects of poisonous bites.

Belladonna should be given if there is any bite from a dog, merely as a precaution against rabies. Also, *Lyssin* (a nosode made from rabies) should also be given if possible, both remedies together, one tablet two times daily for one week. However, conventional anti-rabies injections should be taken if there is any risk of the animal having rabies.

See Chapter Fourteen: Other Tropical and Infectious Diseases, Rabies section

Snake bites
including spiders, scorpions, jelly fish etc.

The effect of snake bites depends partly on the type of snake doing the biting and also the amount of venom that infects the body. The local skin reaction to a snake bite does not necessarily indicate its toxicity. Also, it is not always clear from the wound site if poisoning has actually taken place. Classically the bite marks of a snake are two fang holes, about 1.5 cm or more apart. However, even one fang hole can indicate poisoning. Any wound similar to this needs to be checked and precautions taken (see below). The main physiological action of snake venoms is a hemo-toxic (blood) and neurotoxic (nerves) effect. Overall, most bites from very venomous snakes have a death rate of around 20% if left untreated. The time of the bite till death varies between five hours to two days. At times, with smaller snakes, the wound may not be that obvious and can initially be ignored. However, the smaller snakes may have some of the most virulent poison. It is imperative to get medical help as soon as possible as a precaution. Also take necessary precautions if in an area where poisonous snakes are found. Wear appropriate clothing and shoes, make noise when walking and pay attention. Know the behavior of snakes in the area being visited and find out where and when the greatest risks are.

Most spider bites are not that dangerous and can be treated as any other bites. Occasionally more serious symptoms can develop with occasional fatalities. The most common and quite serious spider bite is from the black widow (Latrodectus mactans), the female of which inflicts the serious bite. They are found in most parts of the world where the weather is warmer. They can often be found under toilet seats in outdoor lavatories and can therefore bite the genitalia. Although the bite itself is hardly felt, within minutes there can be acute symptoms of intense pain in many parts of the body, with spasms through the whole body within an hour. It may seem as if the person is having a heart attack. There may be great difficulty breathing. Symptoms are mostly better within two days. A more severe bite comes from the Sydney funnel web spider (Atrax robustus) which can aggressively pursue its victim and is found in urban areas of Australia. Immediate medical attention is needed with these bites. One spider that creates a necrotic effect of its bite is the brown recluse spider (Loxosceles reclusa). The bite becomes an ulcer, the affected part being 'eaten away' by the venom, leaving much scarring. It can take months to heal. Each of these spiders are homeopathic remedies in their own right but will not be the first line of remedies used. The remedy *Tarentula cubensis* (Cuban spider) can be considered for the ulcerative effects of the funnel web spider as can *Crotalus horridus* and *Lachesis*, both remedies made from snake venom.

Scorpion stings can be very painful and create much local pain and swelling in some cases, but are not as lethal as other bites. However, some scorpions have a more neurotoxic affect and therefore it can have more serious consequences, with symptoms of pain, difficult respiration, sweating and even convulsions.

Jelly fish stings are quite common and are mostly not serious. However, the most serious sting/bite of any creature is from the box jellyfish, found predominantly off the coast of Queensland in the north east of Australia during the summer months, December to July. It is imperative to avoid being stung by these jellyfish. More common is the sting of the Portuguese man-o-war, found in many parts of the world. The sting is intense, with pain and burning of the part. More systemic symptoms can arise, including nausea, vomiting, headache, and a general feeling of shock.

See Shock section and Chapter Twelve: Skin Conditions, Ulcers section

● GENERAL CARE

Clean the wound well, with water, soap and an antiseptic, (*Calendula* tincture, alcohol etc.). Follow with using *Echinacea* tincture to the wound. If the bite is on the arm or leg, tightly bandage the whole limb and keep it still. Do not move unduly. Do not attempt to suck out the poison. If the bite is on another part of the body, clean and apply a bandage, maintaining some pressure on the part if possible. Get medical attention. If a snake bite, the offending snake should be killed so that the appropriate antivenin can be given. The antivenin is made from the venom of the offending snake species. A general antivenin may be given if the identity of the snake is not known. In jelly fish stings, putting vinegar on the sting helps as can urinating on the sting. Also, meat tenderizer can be used on the sting, especially if you prefer that to urine! However, urine may be more immediately accessible!

◆ HOMEOPATHIC CARE

Aconite is the first remedy to give when there is a great emotional shock and fright from the bite. Once the shock has subsided, you can follow on with other remedies. *Lachesis* is the most likely second remedy to give, as described above. *Echinacea* (in tincture or homeopathic potency) can also be given along with or instead of *Lachesis* for the toxic effects of bites, especially when the affected area looks infected and gangrenous. *Apis* is needed when the area is puffy or hard, red, hot and stinging and *Ledum* if the part feels puffy but cold. *Arsenicum album* is needed when there is much burning of the affected part and you feel very chilly and restless and also perhaps feel very anxious and fearful about the situation. In these situations, the remedy needs to be repeated very frequently, between every five to thirty minutes, depending on the severity of symptoms.

COMBINATION STRATEGY If the symptoms are more physical and local, with swelling and red discoloration of the part, begin with *Apis* and also *Ledum*. If it quickly becomes dark blue/purple, give *Lachesis*. If it develops more into looking gangrenous, add *Echinacea*. If burning is predominant, give *Arsenicum album*. If necessary, mix all together in water and take every ten to fifteen minutes for two to three hours. If anxiety and shock are predominant, begin with *Aconite*. Repeat the remedy in water every five minutes for up to one hour. Add *Arsenicum album* if *Aconite* is not enough to relieve the anxiety.

◢ HERBAL CARE

For snake and spider bites, mix clay powder with water to make a clay pack and add a little goldenseal powder or lavender oil. *Echinacea* tincture should be taken internally.

Burns

Burns need to be treated seriously and with great care. It is important to know the degree of severity of the burn, whether it is a first, second or third degree burn. Second and third degree burns often need urgent medical care, especially if a larger area of the body is affected. Any burn which is larger than the size of a hand should have professional medical care. All burns need to be kept clean and free from infection.

● GENERAL CARE

Simple first and second degree burns, affecting a small, local area

Remove any clothing or material that is burning the skin but leave any material that has already been totally burnt. Also leave any dead skin on the burn. Do not peel off. Do not pierce any blisters on second degree burns. Use cool or even slightly warm water to cool the area down. Do not use cold water. (The application of slightly warm water or warm heat may seem contradictory but if done in small frequent applications, it will relieve the burning pain. This is applying the homeopathic law of similars, Like cures Like). If the burn is a second degree, try and soak the burnt part in cool water. Apply homeopathic burn cream or any burn cream once it is dry but not too much to make it too moist. If possible keep the burnt area as still as possible. Ideally do not cover the burn unless there is a risk of infection due to the need to move, travel etc. If so, then place appropriate gauze bandage (non adhesive) loosely to the burnt area and keep in place with a loose bandage. Do not tie too tightly, obstructing the air getting to the burn, which will help it dry and heal. Use the cream frequently to aid the healing process. Also Vitamin E or Aloe vera cream can be used, in conjunction with the burn cream as needed. Egg whites applied to the burn may also be an effective treatment. For sunburn, you can put avocado on the skin to help soothe it. Also coconut oil can be used on the skin, both as a slight sunscreen and also to soothe the skin after the sun. You can also rub coconut meat onto the skin after being in the sun. The sap from an unripe papaya can be used if the burn looks infected, 5 drops of sap and one tablespoon of salt in one liter of boiled water, left to cool.

Second degree burn of a larger area or third degree burn.

Seek medical advice and also use homeopathic remedies as described below. Do not interfere with the burn in any way. Use cool water on the burn area and keep the person still. Using a spray bottle, spray diluted *Calendula* tincture over the burn. Cover the burn with appropriate sterile padding if available or use cling-film or a plastic bag. Do not let the sterile padding or any clothing become dry on the burn area. The plastic helps avoid this and you can wrap moist cloth in plastic if that is what you have. Keep moist (with clean water) until medical attention is found or if in more remote situations and there is no help, then keep a moist padding on the burn area while the pain is intense. Eventually you will have to let the area dry and treat as above for first degree burns. Use damp clothing if no padding is available but again keep it moist to avoid sticking to the burn area.

● HOMEOPATHIC CARE

First degree and simple Second degree burns

Initially *Arnica* can be given for at least two hours (one time every thirty minutes) to address the shock of the burn. Then *Arsenicum album*, *Cantharis* or *Urtica urens* can be given to address the burn. *Cantharis* is the first remedy to consider when you feel intense, burning, scalding pains, and where blisters are forming on the burn. You may feel in an agitated, frenzied state. *Arsenicum album* is needed when you have great anxiety and restlessness with the burning pain. *Urtica urens* is useful in simple first degree burns with little other symptoms.

Second degree (larger area) and Third degree burns.

Aconite is needed immediately after a more serious burn, to address the mental shock. The remedy should be given every five to ten minutes while medical attention is being sought. Once the shock has died down, then *Cantharis* should be given and repeated every thirty minutes for six to eight hours and then less frequently until the pain is under some control. This may take a while. If there are any chronic affects of a more serious burn, especially with feelings of great rawness still in the burnt area, then *Causticum* should be given, once daily for a week. *Radium bromatum* can be considered for burns due to X-rays and other radiation exposure.

🌿 HERBAL CARE

Use some honey with a little lavender oil. Spread liberally over the burn area. Rescue remedy (a Bach flower remedy) can also be taken for the shock. Aloe vera gel is excellent to help relieve sunburn.

Sunburn

Try to avoid getting sunburn. When initially in the sun, pace yourself. Only stay in the sun for short periods at a time. Be aware that you often don't know you are burnt until it is too late. Areas where there is little fat on the body get burnt more quickly. Use good quality sunscreen until you are brown. If you are have pale skin and/or many moles on your body, pay close attention and do not let yourself get burnt. If you notice a mole changing shape, becoming irregular, getting bigger or changing color, get it checked by a doctor.

If you are burnt, get out of the sun. Cool off under a shower but do not use cold water. Use cool water to the burnt part. Once dry, use homeopathic burn cream and/or after-sun lotion. Keep cool and hydrated. If more serious, then treat as for normal burns.

Concussion

Concussion is due to a blow to the head, resulting in some level of confusion and/or temporary unconsciousness. What may seem like a light blow can in fact be concussion. It is important to check to see if there is a possibility for concussion and get medical advice if in doubt. Many people who strike their head say they are fine when they are not.

⬤ GENERAL CARE

If no medical advice is immediately available then sit the person down. Assess if they are confused or not. Look into their eyes. Check to see if one pupil is larger than the other (there may be fluid in the cranial cavity), whether they can follow your finger with their eyes and if they can stand OK. Give them time to recover. Check for headaches, nausea or vomiting, change of pulse or respiration, mental dullness or confusion.

● HOMEOPATHIC CARE

Arnica is the first remedy to give for any concussion. Give one tablet every 30 minutes for at least three hours and wait. If after concussion, there is still some dizziness, confusion and heaviness in the body and the head feels too heavy to hold up, give *Cocculus*. If that doesn't work and there is much trembling of the body and heaviness of the eyelids, give *Gelsemium*.

For chronic complications of a head injury, even years ago, especially if it is chronic headaches or mental depression and anxiety, give *Natrum sulphuricum*, one tablet a day for three days.

Emergencies and Disasters

There are times when some situations become very extreme and out of control and in such intense times, using homeopathic and other natural remedies may literally be a lifesaver. Even when living in fairly safe places, one never knows when something extreme can occur, for example, natural disasters such as tsunamis, floods, fires, earthquakes, volcanoes etc. Or, if witness and exposed to other forms of emergency disasters, e.g., car, boat or plane accidents, extreme violence in war situations, or exposed to toxic chemicals or air pollution e.g., radiation, fire fumes, oil, chemicals in water or the air etc. There are many situations that are out of our control which if we are in the wrong place at the wrong time can profoundly affect us. Knowing which remedies that can be used can be crucial in these times.

● HOMEOPATHIC CARE

For the initial stage of any trauma, two remedies are mostly indicated: *Aconite* and *Arnica*. *Aconite* is for acute mental shock. See Shock section and Chapter Five: Emotional Conditions. *Arnica* is for physical shock. See Accident and Injuries, Concussion, Fractures etc. Both these remedies can be given very frequently, (one tablet dissolved into a glass of water and one sip taken every one to ten minutes) as necessary in acute situations. The more intense the situation, the more frequently the remedy can be taken.

When in a situation where extreme violence is being observed or if one has been threatened by violence, then the same remedies will be used. In extreme situations of intense fear and terror, *Aconite* may often be used with *Stramonium*. See Chapter Five: Emotional Conditions, Fright section. The remedies in the Shock section are also good to know and can also be thought of in any emotional trauma.

In the event of experiencing and surviving a natural disaster like an earthquake, *Aconite* and *Gelsemium* are the two main remedies used for the fear that can remain. If there is a state of collapse or unconsciousness, both from shock or from some physical trauma, *Arnica* is the first remedy but also *Arsenicum album*, *Camphor* and *Carbo veg* are important remedies. See Fainting and Shock sections.

If there has been overexposure to some form of toxic chemical, e.g., radiation, chemicals, chemotherapy or other poisons, then homeopathic remedies can be given. See Poisoning section. *Arsenicum album* is one of the first remedies to consider, especially if there are any burning pains, along with acute restlessness and fear. It is excellent for burns to the skin, or burning of the mouth, esophagus and stomach from ingesting chemicals and for intense nausea from radiation or other chemical poisoning. *Ipecac* is also excellent when chemicals have been ingested, as it helps to purge the body to get rid of the toxicity. *Nux vomica* is also strongly indicated in cases of poisoning when there is much retching, vomiting and spasms in the digestive area. In the case of radiation poisoning, whether from medical radiation or from other forms, *Arsenicum album* is also one of the first remedies. Other remedies include *Radium bromatum* if there is great burning of the skin and of the joints. It is also a remedy for X-ray burns to the skin, along with *Phosphorus*, which also has digestive symptoms from radiation therapy. There is even a homeopathic remedy made from X–ray which can also be used for similar situations and often for chronic skin and organ problems that stem from X-ray exposure. However, constitutional care with a professional is needed in such situations.

Fainting

It is important to know why a person faints. It is due to a lack of blood supply to the brain, and can often happen due to low blood pressure or from emotional stress. It is useful to consult a doctor if it is a recurring condition as some people are more prone to it than others.

● **GENERAL CARE**

If you feel faint, simply sit down and put your head between your knees. Breathe slowly and deeply and wait. Often when stressed, we forget to breathe. If a person has already fainted and is unconscious, simply keep them horizontal, on their side and ensure they have loose clothing and breathing is not impeded. Do not try and rouse them.

● **HOMEOPATHIC CARE**

Aconite is the first remedy to give if fainting is due to any shock, especially sudden and intense fright. *Gelsemium* can also be used if dizziness and trembling are experienced. *Ignatia* should be used if fainting is from emotional shock, such as grief or sudden loss. *Cocculus* is used when fainting is due to lack of sleep and general exhaustion. If fainting arises from too much excitement, then *Ignatia* and also *Coffea* can be given. If it occurs after being angry, then give *Nux vomica*.

Fractures
including dislocation

Most fractures require professional care as soon as possible. Depending on the type of fracture, bones may need to be reset and appropriate structural support given. A fracture is more obvious when the bone is at an unusual angle or there is a distinct shortening of the limb. However, sometimes the break is a compaction and so will not be so obvious. However, the intensity of the pain, bruising and swelling with inability to move very much and pain on any motion may lead to the diagnosis of a fracture.

● GENERAL CARE

In any injury where any movement brings great pain, keep very still and avoid any unnecessary movement. This includes injuries to the spine if there is any chance of a break. In the case where movement is necessary, support the injured part with appropriate measures like an improvised splint or bandaging to minimize motion of the part. You should ideally refer to an appropriate first-aid source for how to do this well.

◆ HOMEOPATHIC CARE

Arnica, ideally in 200c potency can be given straight away, especially if there is much swelling and bruising. If any motion brings great pain, then *Bryonia* should be taken and in this case frequent doses are needed, every fifteen minutes until some relief is felt. It is the first remedy to consider for a dislocation of a joint, along with *Arnica*. The remedies can be alternated if necessary. The remedies should be repeated very frequently as needed. If in a fracture, *Arnica* has been given and there is not much swelling but the pain continues, take *Eupatorium perfoliatum*, one tablet, three times daily for at least three days for the pain. *Symphytum* should be given once the bone has been reset and in place. This can be given once daily for up to two weeks. It will help unite the bone.

Frostbite

Frostbite is due to freezing of parts of the body, usually the extremities and mostly when mountaineering. The frozen part should ideally be thawed slowly if possible. If more serious, then thawing should only be done if refreezing of the part is not going to happen as that can make things worse. Frostbite can also occur at warmer temperatures when the extremities become very wet and also if there is a lack of circulation.

● GENERAL CARE

Any clothing should be dried out as much as possible, including boots. If the part is numb, gentle warmth should be applied, but not excessive heat. If the feet are affected, then ideally you shouldn't be walking far. If the skin breaks, then *Calendula* or *Hypericum* tincture should be added to warm water and a bandage dampened with the warm water mixture and applied to the part.

● HOMEOPATHIC CARE

The remedy *Agaricus muscarius* is a specific remedy to help with frost-bite, including the burning, numbness and tingling often experienced. If that does not work or is not available, then use *Lachesis* instead. Give one tablet four times daily for three to five days.

Hangover

Many people at some time of their life have drunk too much alcohol and suffered the consequences. There is often nausea and/or vomiting and a headache. Mentally there can be great irritability and a desire to stay quiet and alone.

● HOMEOPATHIC CARE

Nux vomica is the most specific remedy for a hangover. It is one of the great remedies for the after effects of alcohol and the classic oversensitivity experienced.

Headache

Headaches are caused by many factors. Headaches of a chronic nature require more constitutional treatment to understand the underlying causes. The only headaches addressed here are due to either trauma, heatstroke, poisoning, including alcohol, and acute emotional states.

● HOMEOPATHIC CARE

Belladonna, *Gelsemium* and *Glonoinum* are the main remedies to consider for headache due to acute heatstroke or any affects from the sun. See Heatstroke section. *Nux vomica* is the remedy to think of for alcohol or other poisoning, *Arnica*, *Cocculus* and *Natrum sulphuricum* if from head trauma. See Concussion sections. *Ignatia* can be thought of if due to acute emotional upset and grief.
See Chapter Five: Emotional Conditions

Heatstroke
including sunstroke and heat exhaustion

Heatstroke (sunstroke) is a condition due to over exposure to sun and often combined with either a lack of fluid intake, excessive alcohol consumption or an inadequate amount of salt in food. It is potentially a very serious condition and can lead to a rapid rise in temperature, nausea, vomiting, collapse and even convulsions. This requires emergency medical intervention.

More commonly found is heat exhaustion, which is not so extreme and occurs from being in the sun too much, and also being dehydrated after exertion. Symptoms often found are dizziness, exhaustion, headache, cramping of muscles, nausea and vomiting. The temperature is much less high than in heatstroke and the person can often feel cool, with shivering. One critical difference between the two is that in heatstroke, the skin tends to be dry and it may be hot and red, whereas in heat exhaustion, it is usually cooler, paler and with more sweat.

Sun headaches are quite common, although some people are much more prone to them than others. The underlying sensitivity to sun exposure requires constitutional homeopathic care.

● **GENERAL CARE**

Due to the increased intensity of the sun, we all have to pay close attention to being over exposed to direct sunlight. It is important to avoid too much exposure. Wearing a hat and keeping hydrated is important. Use good quality sunscreens as necessary. The sun is not bad and some exposure is fine, but in stages and not too much all at once.

In more serious heatstroke cases the person must be put onto the ground if unconscious and bathed with cool sponges. The temperature should not be reduced too quickly. Clothing should be removed and the person ideally covered with a wet sheet and fanned. If conscious, put a damp cloth around the head, neck and extremities. The temperature should be taken frequently, every ten minutes. Once the temperature has lowered to around 103f, this treatment can be stopped. The remedy *Carbo veg* (one tablet put in water, one sip taken every minute) should be given at the same time and *Belladonna* or *Glonoinum* can be followed: see below. Medical attention is necessary.

In heat exhaustion, the person should be allowed to sit or lie down, and to be rehydrated with water and salt (for every half liter, put ½ tsp of salt and four to six tsps of sugar – or in one cup of water, put a pinch of salt and one teaspoon of sugar). Drink slowly and gradually. If you are feeling weak, dizzy, nauseous and not sweating much when in the sun, then take precautionary measures as soon as possible. Rest in the shade for quite a while and rehydrate. Be careful as further exposure to the sun, even days ahead may lead to further problems. Also, be careful with alcohol consumption when in intense heat.

⬥ HOMEOPATHIC CARE

There are two main remedies indicated in heatstroke and acute consequences from being in the sun. The first is *Glonoinum* and the other *Belladonna*. If you need *Glonoinum*, you can experience the most intense throbbing, exploding headache, as if the head is going to blow up. You can feel very hot and flushed and the blood feels as if it is rushing to the head. It is a remedy for extreme congestion of the blood. You can have violent palpitations, which are worse from any motion or jarring. It is the first remedy to think of when there is unconsciousness due to heatstroke. *Belladonna* is the other remedy to consider for such extreme situations but also for simple sun headache when there is heat and throbbing of the head and body. Your pupils can be dilated and you may have a fever, which if very intense, can even include delirium. It is very similar to *Glonoinum*, but *Glonoinum* is even more intense, with more violent congestion.

Gelsemium is very good for sun exhaustion. In this situation, you feel exhausted, achy and dizzy. You can feel confused, disoriented, drowsy and chilled, often with trembling. See Shock section.

Hemorrhage

Hemorrhage is any form of unnatural bleeding. It is important to know the reason why a hemorrhage is occurring and to seek professional medical care if there are any doubts. The following remedies can be considered for different kinds of hemorrhage and can even be given while on the way to getting medical care.

See Chapter Ten Women's Conditions, After Birth section

● HOMEOPATHIC CARE

Arnica is the first remedy for any hemorrhage due to injury e.g., nosebleed or from any other orifice. There can be great bruising of the skin and soreness. *Hamamelis* is another remedy for bleeding which can be used if *Arnica* doesn't work. It is great for bleeding hemorrhoids and bleeding gums after tooth extraction and nosebleeds after a blow. The flow of blood is often dark, persistent and may be oozing.

Ipecac is a remedy for any bleeding associated with nausea, especially uterine bleeding of any sort, particularly after childbirth or miscarriage. It is also used for nosebleeds with coughing and nausea. The blood is often bright red and profuse. *Phosphorus* can also be given when bleeding occurs very easily, again with bright red blood and like *Ipecac* is needed after childbirth or from uterine fibroids. *Belladonna* is useful for any bleeding where the blood is bright red and hot and the face feels hot and red with a pulsating pulse. *China* is good when bleeding is associated with fainting and weakness. It may be from the uterus or from the rectum with diarrhea. *Mercurius* is useful for bleeding from the rectum with diarrhea

See Chapter Six : Digestive Conditions, Dysentery section

● HERBAL CARE

Shepherds Purse (*Thlaspi bursa pastoris*) tincture to 6x. For uterine hemorrhage, with cramps and colic, whether from a miscarriage, labor and post labor. Follow instructions on the label on how to take if in a tincture. If in a homeopathic potency, take one tablet three to five times daily for two days.

See Chapter Ten: Women's conditions

Jetlag

This is a common condition that most people experience to some extent. Some people however are much more affected by it than others and if so, it is good to take some remedies preventatively to minimize symptoms. Altering one's watch to read the time at the destination may help to relieve jetlag!

● GENERAL CARE

When flying, it is important to keep hydrated and to minimize alcohol content. Dehydration is a major factor in jetlag, especially in long haul flights. Drink a lot of liquid. Also put a little more salt on your food and/or take rehydration salts. It is important to keep moving during long haul flights to stop the possibility of deep vein thrombosis.

● HOMEOPATHIC CARE

Arnica can be taken three times the day before the flight for general preparation if you experience jetlag normally. *Cocculus* can also be given in this way if you feel the following symptoms from jetlag – weakness, heaviness and dizziness and even hollowness in the body, especially the head. *Cocculus* is one of the great remedies for problems from a loss of sleep, and if you suffer a lot from losing sleep, then this remedy is indicated. *Nux vomica* is for when you feel as if you are hung over, feeling oversensitive to noise and feeling irritable and touchy.

NOTE You can take whichever picture most fits your experience with jetlag, even just before flying. You can also often find a combination homeopathic remedy called NoJetLag at airport shops and take that if you have no other remedies.

Pain

It is important to find out the reasons for any pain. There are good homeopathic remedies for a variety of pains and will be found discussed in the regions affected or the conditions associated with the pain. It is important to know exactly what the pain feels like and how the person, even if it is you, is dealing with the pain. Do you want to keep still, move around, shriek, weep or become angry with the pain? This makes a difference which remedy may be needed. As always, getting professional care can be important to understand what is going on.

● HOMEOPATHIC CARE

Chamomilla is one of the great remedies for pain used in homeopathy, especially in children. Pains seem unendurable, with much crying, even shrieking and anger. This is seen in abdominal colic, teething pain and fever. It is as if the reaction is well beyond what it should be. *Coffea* is another pain remedy, especially teeth pain but also colic and other pains. There can be great oversensitivity, and great restlessness and weeping with the pain. *Nux vomica* is also similar to both these remedies and the pain is intense, cramping and spasmodic, and seen with anger, intolerance and great sensitivity.

Bryonia is a great pain remedy, especially for broken bones and injuries where the slightest motion creates intense sharp and bursting pain. *Hypericum* is the remedy needed for nerve pains, especially injuries to nerve rich areas, e.g., fingers being trapped in doors, lacerations to nerve areas, back injuries etc. Pains are sharp, shooting, violent, feeling intolerable. *Arnica* is the remedy given when the pains always feel sore, as if bruised.

Colocynthis is excellent for acute abdominal colic, doubling the person up and needing to put great pressure into the abdomen. It is the remedy when colic comes on after suppressed anger. *Magnesium phosphoricum* is very similar and a great remedy for all spasmodic pains, colic and cramping pains, all of which come on suddenly and which change place frequently. There are neuralgic pains better from heat and pressure, including toothache and colic. Pains can extort cries. The person can be constantly talking about their pains.

Poisoning

● **GENERAL CARE**

At times, accidental poisonings occur, either due to intake of toxic chemicals (something children can do inadvertently) and also by eating poisonous mushrooms and other plants. Medical intervention is ideally required, especially if the toxic dose is large or the person is becoming unconscious. It is very useful to know what type of poison has been taken. In general, the poison needs to be purged from the body and an emetic can be given to do this. Salt and warm water will work well, using at least one tablespoon of salt to a large glass of water. It should be drunk quickly to encourage frequent vomiting. If it is mushroom poisoning, then salt and water should not be given but vomiting should be induced with an emetic like *Ipecac*. Also some of the mushroom species ingested should be collected for examination later. If the poisons are corrosive chemicals, then emetics should not be used but alkaline liquids given such as Milk of Magnesia can be taken.

Other forms of poisoning include the ingestion of chemicals and also the after effects of conventional medicine, in the form of chemo-therapy and radiation. Remedies can be given to help in such situations. Miso soup has been known to be effective in helping to detoxify from exposure to radiation. Japanese people have been using this method.

◆ **HOMEOPATHIC CARE**

If there is intense vomiting and purging already taking place, then give *Arsenicum album*. This can be followed by *Veratrum album* if there is cold sweat on the forehead. If the person is in a state of collapse, then *Carbo veg* should be given. See Shock section. *Aconite* can be given if there is a lot of anxiety and fear. However, professional care should be sought as soon as possible.

In cases where toxic drugs have been taken, including the use of chemotherapy for cancer, then *Arsenicum album* is one of the first reme-dies when there is great nausea and burning pains in the body, especially in the digestive sphere. *Sepia* and *Tabacum* are two other important remedies when extreme nausea is felt. In *Sepia* there is nausea which is much worse from the smell and taste of food but also can be better after eating food. In *Tabacum* there is intense nausea with a sinking and deathly feeling, a cold sweat and at times a collapsed state.

Shock

Shock can be either physical or mental. Both issues are dealt with here. This also includes situations when a person has collapsed. In mental shock, the person is normally conscious but often in a state that includes profound agitation, disorientation, confusion, fear with shaking, rapid heart- beat and dizziness etc. The cause of the shock can be varied, from being in or seeing an accident, or an earthquake or some other natural trauma or disaster; or from experiencing violence, both verbal and physical, or anything sudden and extremely intense.

See Concussion, Fainting and Heatstroke sections and Chapter Five: Anxiety and Grief

● **GENERAL CARE**

Physical shock or collapse may come from simply fainting or it can be due to more serious and intense physical conditions, such as a heart attack. It may also be due to a loss of blood or the affects of physical trauma. Often the person is either semi-conscious or unconscious. In either case, the first thing to do is to take care of the person. They need to be placed in a horizontal position on one side and to ensure they can breathe freely. If the person is not breathing, then resuscitation should be given. (A first aid course should be taken to gain the necessary knowledge of this). Professional medical care should be sought.

◆ **HOMEOPATHIC CARE**

Aconite is the first remedy to give for any acute mental shock when great fear and anxiety are seen. *Arnica* is given for any physical shock due to physical trauma, especially concussion to the head. If conscious, a person can say he is fine even when not fine or does not want to be touched. Other remedies may follow in head injury, including *Hypericum* and *Natrum sulphuricum*. *Opium* is also a remedy for extreme emotional shock and fright, and is similar to *Aconite*. Both remedies are indicated if one has witnessed a terrible accident or experienced war trauma.

Carbo veg is useful for any state of collapse with blueness of the face and difficulty breathing. People can look lifeless. There is often a need for fresh air and being fanned, even if already outside, although they may feel cold and have cold breath. The pulse may be imperceptible. General weakness from any shock is seen. *Camphor* is needed in similar conditions of collapse with great icy coldness as a result of shock. Even though cold, they may not want to be covered. Both remedies are needed if someone collapses from diarrhea, along with *Arsenicum album* and *Veratrum album*.

Ignatia is the remedy for emotional shock and grief, when there is sudden bad news, loss, disappointment or grief. Emotionally there is a distraught state with sobbing and sighing, or an inability to cry, even if there is a desire to. There can be spasms and twitching of the body in the shock state and even unconsciousness, which *Aconite*, *Chamomilla* and *Coffea* also can have. *Gelsemium* is also good for shock when there is confusion, sleepiness, a heaviness of the body and the eyelids feel heavy with a desire to fall asleep. There can be great anxiety and trembling remaining after the shock.

COMBINATION STRATEGY In any state of sudden collapse, you can combine *Arsenicum album*, *Camphor* and *Carbo veg* if the picture isn't clear. *Aconite* and *Opium* can be combined if there is extreme fear remaining after a shock

Sleeplessness

Sleeplessness can be caused by many factors. Sometimes it is a chronic ongoing condition and in that case, constitutional homeopathic treatment is needed. In more acute situations, it is mostly due to anxiety, jetlag, or because of another physical condition being experienced. There are many allopathic and herbal options to help with sleep, including sleeping tablets, melatonin (if available) and various herbal and homeopathic formulas. The following homeopathic remedies are suggested for simple occasional sleeplessness.

Cocculus is a good remedy when after having missed sleep, it is difficult to relax and fall asleep. This can happen when traveling overnight or when very little sleep has been had for days. It is also excellent for states of anxiety and worry that come from the stress of travel, or looking after people and feeling overwhelmed. Often you can feel heavy, tired, dizzy and confused. *Chamomilla* and *Coffea* are two other good remedies to consider. In *Chamomilla*, which is excellent for children, there is great agitation, frustration and anger. Children just cannot be pacified, nothing will relieve them. It is good to give just before sleep. In *Coffea*, there is great over excitability, restlessness and the mind feels it is working too hard. It is good when there are many things on your mind, perhaps anticipating events and simply unable to relax.

Nux vomica is also excellent and similar to *Chamomilla* and *Coffea*. There is great nervousness, irritation and even anger, a wound up, touchy state. It is the remedy to give if sleeplessness comes from drinking too much alcohol. *Ignatia* should be given when you feel you can't sleep from grief, worry and anxiety, when you feel sad and weepy and your moods are changeable and erratic.

● HERBAL CARE

Valeriana in a tea form or tincture can be given to help aid sleep.

Spinal (Back) Injury

● GENERAL CARE

In any injury to the back, it is important to know how serious the injury is. It is important to keep still initially in evaluating the nature of the injury. If the injury involves a break to the back, then undue movement may lead to paralysis or at least a complication of the situation. Nerves may be involved in back injuries. If the injury seems serious, then wait until the shock has died down before moving. If less serious, still be careful. If the injury is to the coccyx, it may be broken. Seeing a doctor for a diagnosis can be very important to get an idea of the severity of the injury.

If the injury does not seem severe and there is a simple jolt or shock to the spine, you should begin with *Arnica*, giving one tablet three times a day for two days. *Hypericum* can then be given to follow for two days. *Hypericum* is especially indicated for injuries to the coccyx when there are shooting pains and difficulty in sitting. For injuries to the neck, including whiplash, *Arnica* should first be given, followed by *Hypericum*. If there is residual dizziness or nausea, the head feels heavy and there is mental confusion, then give *Gelsemium*. If that doesn't finish it, give *Cocculus*. If mental confusion remains or generally you do not feel normal, even months or years after the injury take *Natrum sulphuricum*, one tablet daily for three days.

For more general injuries to the back due to straining and over lifting, then *Arnica* should be given first for one to two days, followed by *Rhus tox* or *Ruta grav*, especially if there is stiffness in the back with difficulty to straighten up when rising from sitting. There can be spasms of pain after injury, especially after exposure to cold and damp weather and pains are better from pressure and warmth. *Nux vomica* can follow if the spasms are not fully relieved. *Ledum* is indicated when pains from a strain vary in their position and also come with great stiffness. However, pains are often worse from heat, the opposite of *Rhus tox*, *Ruta grav* and *Nux vomica*. *Chamomilla* is good when the pains seem intolerable, forcing one from bed and pacing the floor. The pain induces a lot of anger, similar to *Nux vomica*.

Sprains

A sprain to a joint, often the ankle, knee or wrist can be debilitating and very painful initially and greatly limiting if traveling. It can also be difficult to distinguish from a break and a medical evaluation is often needed to confirm the diagnosis.

● GENERAL CARE

Ensure the injured part is supported well with an appropriate bandage. Follow good first aid care. Be careful to rest the part as much as possible but if it is not broken, then gradual gentle motion is good. Use topical treatment of *Arnica* cream and/or *Rhus tox* cream on the injured part. Try not to re-injure the part by using it too much. Check with a doctor to see if it is only a sprain or whether a bone may be broken if pain continues.

● HOMEOPATHIC CARE

Arnica is the first remedy to give for the basic trauma, especially if there is bruising and swelling to the area and it is worse for touch. It should then be followed by another remedy depending on the symptoms. *Bryonia* should be given when it is excruciatingly painful, and is worse for any movement, touch and jar. There is a need to keep the injured part very still. *Rhus tox* is good when there is great stiffness in the injured area and pain on initial movement, but which then gets better from continued motion and also at times by warmth. *Ruta grav* is similar to *Rhus tox* and is especially indicated in injuries to wrists, tennis elbow and small joints, as well as the shin area, where the periosteum is involved. *Ledum* follows *Arnica* well when the part remains bruised and swollen, in spite of *Arnica* and especially if the injured part feels cold.

Surgery

All forms of surgery are traumatic events for the body and mind and some homeopathic remedies can be helpful in overcoming the trauma involved.

● HOMEOPATHIC CARE

Arnica is the first remedy to consider for any surgery, including having teeth extracted or operated on. Give one tablet three times the day before any surgery and then three times daily for up to three days after. *Bellis perennis* is to be given if surgery is on deep abdominal tissue, often leaving the person feeling very sore and bruised. *Staphysagria* is good when there are lacerated wounds, due to surgical incision, especially in very sensitive areas such as the abdomen or genitalia. Often the wound feels very sensitive and there can be a feeling of violation and great over-sensitivity. *Calendula* can be used in a tincture and applied locally as well as in a homeopathic potency if the wound of the surgery is very painful. See Wounds section. Also look at remedies in the Shock section if there is shock involved. If the surgery required general anesthetic and the person is having a hard time recovering from this, feeling spacey and disoriented, then *Phosphorus* can be given three times daily for up to three days. If nausea remains after anesthetic, give *Arsenicum album* and follow with *Nux vomica* is that doesn't work.

Travel Sickness

Travel sickness is a common affliction but which can be very debilitating. Some people get it much worse than others and if that is the case, preventative care should be taken, both conventionally and homeopathically. If you know of a homeopathic remedy that has worked before, then this should be taken before you travel.

● HOMEOPATHIC CARE

Tabacum is the first remedy to consider for serious travel sickness, especially sea sickness. There is often a deathly nausea, your face has a white pallor with cold perspiration and you often feel a great sinking feeling in the stomach. There can be weakness and trembling and even a feeling like you might even die. Any tobacco smoke makes symptoms worse. *Cocculus* has nausea, vomiting, dizziness and weakness due to movement of a boat or car. You are unable to look at any moving object and the nausea is worse at the sight or smell of food. Symptoms are better when lying down and worse when sitting up and raising the head. *Nux vomica* has violent nausea, gagging and retching but you are unable to fully expel vomit. *Borax* can be useful in travel sickness due to sudden downward motion.

COMBINATION STRATEGY If in doubt, take one tablet of every remedy, mixing in water and taking one tsp. every five to ten minutes until there is relief or simply take in tablet form.

Wounds

● GENERAL CARE

Any wound in which the skin is broken needs to be cleaned and protected from infection. Be very attentive of even small wounds in the tropics, especially around the feet. Clean well and cover if possible. General first aid care with use of band aids and bandages need to be used and homeopathic care used to supplement this. Carry *Calendula* tincture and tea tree oil for basic disinfectant. If a wound is deep, due to a nail or other pointed object, try and get the wound to bleed. This is to prevent tetanus which can only grow where there is no oxygen. Once a wound is dressed, it can be left for days until the wound is somewhat healed. The dressing should not be changed. Even if the wound continues to weep, do not change it daily, only when totally necessary. Spray *Calendula* tincture onto the bandage which will maintain the disinfectant of the wound. Internal homeopathic remedies can be given along with local applications. Plain sugar can also be put on a wound and then dressed with a bandage.

See Chapter Sixteen: Prevention, Tetanus

● HOMEOPATHIC CARE

Calendula in a homeopathic tincture can be used to wash and clean any wound, including a puncture wound, ulcer and laceration. Some tincture should be put into warm water and the injured area cleaned thoroughly. It should be followed by *Calendula* or Hyper/cal cream or ointment. It is imperative to thoroughly clean a puncture wound to prevent infection. Tea tree oil and/or lavender oil can be used topically instead of or along with the *Calendula* and *Hypericum*.

Calendula can be given in a 30c potency for lacerated wounds, especially if very painful. *Ledum* is given for punctured wounds with *Hypericum* to follow in injury to nerve rich areas with sharp shooting pains. *Staphysagria* is needed for painful lacerations, especially in vulnerable areas, e.g., abdomen, around the eyes, genitalia etc. There is a great feeling of violation, emotional sensitivity and vulnerability. *Silicea* is useful for splintered wounds, in order to help extract the splinter or spines in the skin.

Chapter Five
Emotional Conditions

If you are feeling anxious, angry or any other emotional stress, breathing slowly and deeply can help. Often we forget to do this and it can greatly relieve anxiety by using breathing to calm down. There is a type of breathing in yoga where you contract the back of the throat, narrowing the passages for air, allowing more control of both inhalation and exhalation. It is called ujjayi breath and it can greatly help when emotions of all sorts threaten to overwhelm. You can use this method to breathe slowly but deeply for a few minutes but the main thing is to use the breath to calm down and to gain control of strong emotions.

Strong emotional feelings can come up at any time and for many reasons and in homeopathy it can be an important part of understanding what remedy may be useful, both for physical conditions and also to deal with intense emotional states that may arise, whether traveling or simply in one's daily life.

Anger

Anger that exists out of proportion to a situation is something to be very aware of. In cultures where anger is not appropriate or when faced with situations that are very stressful, one has to cultivate great restraint. Homeopathic treatment should be given if this is a common occurrence or when there are physical and/or emotional consequences from becoming angry. If anger is a common reaction to situations, then constitutional homeopathic care or some form of therapy should be taken.

◗ HOMEOPATHIC CARE

If anger comes after an experience of being humiliated or treated badly and you feel indignant, frustrated and feel unable to express these feelings, then two remedies are often indicated, *Colocynthis* and *Staphysagria*. With *Staphysagria*, you often feel very oversensitive, even weepy, and often very humiliated. You may not even feel angry, more simply upset, or you can feel a great anger with a desire to throw things or break things. You feel very frustrated. In *Colocynthis*, similar feelings are also experienced, often along with great cramping, especially in the abdomen, the pains even doubling you up and you want to press deeply into the abdomen for relief. With both remedies, the initial anger is suppressed and then other symptoms arise, both physical and psychological. Anger may come up later, along with great indignation.

Nux vomica is needed if you have feelings of pent up wrath, feeling extremely touchy and sensitive to all impressions, including noises, smells etc. You feel very intolerant and impatient and it takes a lot of energy to contain your anger. *Chamomilla* is needed when capriciousness and rage are felt and you just don't know what you want to do. You feel really frustrated, touchy, impatient and intolerant, but not so full of rage as when you need *Nux vomica*. *Chamomilla* is great for angry children who throw everything they are given and cannot be placated in anyway.

Anxiety

Anxiety exists for many reasons and may often be utterly appropriate to the situation. Anticipatory anxiety is also common when traveling or before exams. It should not be treated unless it does not go away or seems extreme for the situation at hand.

◆ HOMEOPATHIC CARE

If anxiety is felt as a result of an extreme shock or fright, then *Aconite* is the first remedy to consider. If you have felt any deep shock, even as extreme as feeling as if you could die, e.g., being in or even watching an accident, then take *Aconite*. If you feel more anticipatory anxiety or have experienced a shock which makes you tremble and very apprehensive, as if you are waiting to experience the same thing again, then *Gelsemium* is the remedy. *Gelsemium* is the first remedy for all kinds of anticipatory anxiety, even to having diarrhea. This is a great remedy to have for all kinds of travel based anxiety.

If you feel anxiety as if you are wired up on coffee and you feel oversensitive to everything, including noises, smells and any stimulus then homeopathic *Coffea* is the remedy. This is an example of how homeopathy works. Like Cures Like. *Coffea* is an excellent remedy for anxiety states, especially when you feel very tense, agitated or impatient and your mind is racing very fast.

◢ HERBAL CARE

Valeriana can be taken for nervous anxiety and sleeplessness. Rescue remedy (A Bach Flower Remedy) can also be taken for any kind of shock and anxiety. It can be used along with a homeopathic remedy and you can take it as often as feels needed when anxiety arises.

Fright

Acute fright can be experienced at any time. Unpredictable events can occur at any time and the shock involved can leave a lasting effect.
See Chapter Four: Accidents, Injuries and Trauma, Anxiety and Shock sections

● GENERAL CARE

If you experience or see a person experiencing a fright do nothing until you feel the shock diminish. Sit down and breathe deeply. If the fright continues then take one of the homeopathic remedies.

Aconite and *Gelsemium* are the two main remedies to consider, similar to anxiety, and their symptom picture is described above in the anxiety section and elsewhere. Both *Gelsemium* and *Aconite* are good after experiencing an earthquake or similar type of trauma. *Stramonium* is a very good remedy for ailments from fright when great fear and terror remain, and also has a strong fear of the dark, of being alone at night and of dogs. It is one of the main remedies when extreme fear is due to any violence seen or experienced. *Opium* is needed when great fear remains after experiencing or witnessing a terrible event, e.g., accident, war trauma etc. In *Opium* you feel as if frozen in the fear, a 'fear of fear' and the only escape is to become emotionally numb, cut off from your feelings. You need *Cocculus* when you feel weak, dizzy and dull after a fright. There is great heaviness and similar to *Gelsemium*, the head can feel too heavy to hold up. You can also take Rescue Remedy, 3 drops, every 15-60 minutes until you feel relief. Take it as necessary along with a homeopathic remedy.

Grief

Grief is a normal reaction to emotional trauma but at times it is hard to overcome. Taking homeopathic remedies is useful to help any state of grief.

⬥ HOMEOPATHIC CARE

Ignatia is the first remedy to think of for any grief, be it romantic loss, or the death of a close friend or family member. The feeling is one of shock and an inability to reconcile the grief. Emotionally you can feel as if you want to cry but can't, or can't stop crying. Sobbing may be uncontrollable with much sighing and even cramping in parts of the body. You may feel a lump in the throat and a choking feeling, making it difficult to swallow. Your moods are changing all the time. *Natrum muriaticum* often follows *Ignatia* and is needed when there is a feeling of sadness and grief but with no weeping. You feel you want to weep but simply can't express the feelings. Everything is held in. You want to be alone and think of the grief, but that doesn't help. You may listen to sad music which makes the sadness worse but you don't want to share it with anybody.

Cocculus is needed when there is great sadness, heaviness and weakness. You may feel like you can't sleep at night and in the day you feel just dazed and unable to focus on anything else. It is as if you are in your own world. *Pulsatilla* is needed if you feel deserted, forsaken and lost. You can have much weepiness and feel unable to control your emotions. Your moods change all the time and there is a great desire for company and consolation, or where at times you really want to be alone and then later really want to be in company. Your moods are very changeable.

The Natural Medicine Guide For Travel And Home

Chapter Six
Digestive Conditions

Abdominal Pain

It is important to know if abdominal problems, especially pain which is very intense, could be due to appendicitis, pelvic inflammatory disease, menstrual problems, gall bladder problems, inflammation of the pancreas or spleen, liver problems or obstruction of the intestines. Some pain can also be referred from the back, perhaps due to kidney problems or structural back problems. If pain persists, see a medical practitioner for a diagnosis.

See Constipation, Diarrhea, Dysentery, Food poisoning, Heartburn, Hepatitis, Indigestion sections. Also see Chapter Ten: Women's Conditions

Appendicitis

Appendicitis is an inflammation of the appendix, a small protrusion found in the small intestine. Appendicitis often requires surgery because if the appendix bursts, it can lead to a more generalized infection of the whole body (peritonitis), which can be life threatening. It is very important to get a medical diagnosis if there is any doubt about any abdominal pain. It is not always easy to diagnose. The classic area of pain is in the right lower half of the abdomen, two to three inches in from the hip joint. Pain is often better when pressure is applied but then gets much worse when pressure is released suddenly. Sometimes, pain can initially be felt more in the navel (umbilical) region and radiates from there. If pain begins there for no apparent reason and doesn't go away in 24 hours, press into the appendix region to see if there is any sensitivity there. If in doubt, get a medical diagnosis.

● **GENERAL CARE**

As with any inflammation, drink more water. Do not do any strenuous exertions. Relax and rest. Do not eat anything for 24 hours and see if that makes a difference. If in doubt, take one of the homeopathic remedies and head for the nearest emergency room hospital.

◆ **HOMEOPATHIC CARE**

Bryonia is the first remedy to consider for appendicitis. You may experience an intense pain either in the lower right quadrant of the abdomen or in the umbilical area and any movement makes the pain worse. You want to keep very still. Putting pressure on the painful area may make the pain better and any jarring makes it worse. *Belladonna* is the second remedy to think of, especially if you feel the pain come on very suddenly and intensely, the pain being bursting, sharp and/or throbbing. You may have a high burning fever, which is higher and more intense than felt in the *Bryonia* picture. With both remedies there may be increased thirst.

Arnica may also be needed if there is a bruised, sore feeling in the appendix region and you don't want the area touched, but *Bryonia* should be given first and if necessary followed by one of the other remedies. If the remedy is correct, a change should be seen within one to three hours. The remedy should be taken ideally in liquid, one tsp. every five to ten minutes.

✿ **HERBAL CARE**

Take *Echinacea* tincture, 30 drops, hourly for one day.

Colic

Colic is painful contractions of parts of the body, most often felt in the abdomen (intestines) and also in the kidneys and ureters (tubes from the kidney to bladder) and the bile duct near the liver. Abdominal colic is often seen in young babies and children when they are having difficulty digesting milk or food. Symptoms are extremely painful contractions of the affected part, making the person double up in pain and the pain comes in spasms. Often you want to grab the painful part and keep it still or put much pressure onto it.

See Chapter Eleven: Bladder and Kidney

● **GENERAL CARE**

It is good to allow the person to lie down in whichever position they want and just give support. Having this type of pain can be very unsettling. If it is kidney colic, it may indicate stones in the kidney and urinary tract which may require medical intervention.

◗ **HOMEOPATHIC CARE**

The first remedy to consider for abdominal colic is *Colocynthis*. The pain is as if the abdomen is twisting and cutting, or as if it is being squeezed between two stones. There can be great restlessness and wanting to bend double and to press very intensely into the abdomen. It can also be indicated in colic of the kidneys. It is excellent when colic comes after a bout of anger or indignation, similar to that of *Staphysagria*. If anger is the precipitating cause and *Colocynthis* doesn't work, give *Staphysagria*. *Chamomilla* is the first remedy to consider for colic in babies, when there is much screaming and weeping and the child wants to be carried all the time. *Nux vomica* is a good remedy for all sorts of colic, intestinal as well as kidney and liver, especially if from over indulging in rich food or alcohol. There can be great irritability with the symptoms. *Bryonia* is good when you want to stay very still with the pains. Every movement makes it worse and staying still is the best thing to do. *Berberis* is useful particularly in kidney (renal) colic, especially when the pain is spreading out in waves to the rest of the body. *Magnesium phosphoricum* can be given if *Colocynthis* is indicated but doesn't work or where the symptoms are much better from warm or hot applications to the abdomen as well as bending double. *Lycopodium* has colic associated with liver and gall bladder issues, often seen with abdominal swelling and much gas being passed. There is a great aversion to clothing around the waist. It can be given in kidney colic when the right kidney is affected.

See Chapter Eleven: Bladder and Kidney

Constipation

This can be due to many reasons. It is important to investigate any possible mechanical causes for constipation, especially in young children. Hemorrhoids may also be a cause of constipation. Mostly, constipation is a chronic condition that requires more constitutional treatment. However, when 'on the road' constipation can be a frequent problem, due to dietary differences and also due to being unable or reluctant to go in strange places. One should seek medical attention if the constipation persists for more than five days without any bowel movement or is associated with much rectal bleeding, weight loss or frequent intense pain in the intestines.

See Hemorrhoids section

● GENERAL CARE

Keep hydrated. Drink enough water, wherever you are. If you need to make a rehydration mixture, use one teaspoon of salt with eight teaspoons of sugar and one liter of clean water. Eat food that encourages bowel function – fresh fruit, vegetables, and especially prunes or figs. Ensure you get enough roughage in your diet, and ideally whole grains. Avoid too much white rice.

◆ HOMEOPATHIC CARE

Nux vomica is the best remedy to take for simple constipation on the road. You can feel a frequent urging but very little or nothing comes out. This may also be associated with painful hemorrhoids. You may also feel quite irritable with the constipation and a feeling of being unfinished after a stool. *Bryonia* can also be given when the stool seems very dry and there is a general dryness of the whole body, especially the mouth and lips.

🍃 HERBAL CARE

Take probiotics with you when you travel to help maintain a healthy flora in your intestines. Ground flax seeds or Chia seeds can be used and also psyllium is very useful for constipation as well as diarrhea.
See Diarrhea section

Diaper (Nappy) Rash

This is a condition where there is inflammation around the anus, leading to redness and at times rawness, pain and great discomfort. There can be infections in the area, mainly bacterial or fungal in origin.

● GENERAL CARE

Allow the area to be open to the air as much as possible. Ensure diapers are changed frequently. Wash the area thoroughly and dry very well. Use a good cream, such as homeopathic *Calendula* cream (especially if more infected) or baby powder. Breast milk can be used as well.

◆ HOMEOPATHIC CARE

When the child's anus is very red with great burning and a fever is involved, give *Belladonna*. If the child is screaming inconsolably and it feels nothing gives relief give *Chamomilla*. *Rhus tox* is excellent when there are weeping blisters and great redness with restlessness.

🍃 HERBAL CARE

Use *Calendula* cream.

Diarrhea

Diarrhea is one of the most frequent experiences of travelers. Often due to eating bad food or water and/or infections with viruses, bacteria or amoebas, diarrhea is the natural reaction of the body to purge the offending bugs. Suppressing diarrhea should only be done when absolutely necessary and should not be a routine event when diarrhea ensues. Antibiotics such as Cipro should not be given in the first few days of diarrhea before it is known what type of diarrhea one has. Use natural methods first. While most cases of diarrhea are self-limiting (up to 80% clear up on their own in three days) some can become more serious conditions and need to be treated effectively. Do not immediately take drugs to bung you up (Imodium, Lomotil etc.) if you get a dose of diarrhea. Let nature take its course unless you have to travel and could find yourself in trouble. Normally the body has to purge the toxins from the system. Taking these medications simply prevents your body doing what it needs to do. They can also cause complications if you have dysentery or have any blood in your stool. Also do not give them to children. Give some rehydration salts/powders and wait it out.

If taking conventional drugs, ensure they are what they say they are and are safe. Many drugs found in the developing world can be unsafe, or have been banned in other countries. Seek appropriate medical advice for diagnosis and treatment. Any lingering diarrhea that continues after travel has to be checked out by a medical specialist for diagnostic purposes. Do not ignore lingering symptoms, especially after travel to 'exotic' places.

One of the most common infections is giardiasis, a protozoa which can be easily caught both in tropical and temperate climates. It is less acute than other infectious diarrheas but tends to last much longer, often with weakness, fullness and very offensive fatty stools. At times it only begins once back from a vacation due to an incubation period of over one week. Having a stool test can be useful to confirm diagnosis. However, homeopathic treatment should be commenced immediately. The most specific remedy for it is *China*. Also See Dysentery section. Treatment should be given for at least one week. Be patient. Improvement will begin between one to three days but will take longer to fully get better. The remedy should be taken three times a day.

Cholera is historically one of the most intense and dangerous diarrheal diseases but today, for most travelers and in developed societies, it is rarely seen. It occurs most commonly in times and places where hygiene and clean water is severely lacking and many people are living together in cramped circumstances, e.g., war situations and other natural traumas. It is a bacterial disease and is spread through contaminated water and food. Some people can be carriers of the disease and once infected, the incubation period is normally between two to seven days.

See Chapter Fifteen: Other Tropical and Infectious Diseases, Cholera

Diarrhea can also be associated with other conditions, including malaria and typhoid. If diarrhea comes with a fever, consider these conditions. If there is fever and blood in the stool, consider bacillary dysentery, but if there's blood in the stool with no fever, it may be amoebic dysentery. Bilharzia/Schistosomiaisis may also have blood in stool and also urine with no fever. If diarrhea is extremely severe, like rice water, but no blood is seen and no fever, consider cholera.

See Chapter Fourteen: Other Tropical and Infectious Conditions, Bilharzia

Liver flukes may be another reason for diarrhea, often associated in the acute phase with nausea and abdominal pain. More long term symptoms include fatigue, weight loss, abdominal discomfort, jaundice and anorexia. They can affect liver and bile duct function and other more chronic conditions can ensue. They are often caught from eating undercooked fish and are particularly prevalent in Far East Asia. It can be tested for and conventional treatment is available.

● GENERAL CARE

As a prevention, ensure the food you eat is well cooked, especially meat. Drink only water that has been well boiled and purified or use bottled water.

See Chapter Three: Being Prepared, Food and Water section.

Once you have diarrhea, avoid milk, meat, fatty, spicy and any other irritating foods. Keep to a simple diet or simply do not eat for 24-48 hours. Bananas are OK but avoid citrus fruit. If you feel hungry, plain white rice with a little plain yoghurt is good or just rice and other dry foods – bread, toast, etc. Keep hydrated by drinking good water and if dehydration is suspected, introduce some re-hydration ingredients with the water.

Tea made from neem and artemesia leaves may relieve diarrhea and also tea from leaves of the guava and mango tree can be effective (1 tablespoon of pounded leaves each). The latter can be mixed together and is good for amoebic dysentery. Although fruit in general should be avoided, eating ripe mangoes can also help in amoebic dysentery.

🔴 HOMEOPATHIC CARE

The first remedy to consider in acute diarrhea of all sorts is *Arsenicum album*. It is excellent for all food poisoning. Diarrhea can be very acute, with great burning when passing stool and you may also have nausea and vomiting with it. Often you may feel exhausted after passing stool. You may feel worse at the sight or smell of food and are often chilled.

Two other commonly needed remedies are *Podophyllum* and *Veratrum album*. The latter remedy often looks like *Arsenicum album*, with nausea and/or vomiting along with the diarrhea, but it has more chill and cold perspiration with the stool, especially on the forehead. *Podophyllum* has very characteristic rumbling and gurgling in the abdomen, often just before stool, which then comes out in a violent intense, explosive gush. There can also be involuntary stool, especially at night. The stool can be either very odorous or doesn't smell at all.

If diarrhea is experienced with intense cramping pains in the abdomen, then *Colocynthis* and *Nux vomica* should be looked at. In *Colocynthis*, it feels as if the intestines are being twisted or squeezed and the pain forces you to bend double and/or to press intensely into the abdomen. *Nux vomica* also can have intense cramping, often just before stool, and the urging is intense and nearly always unsatisfying. There can also be spasmodic nausea, retching and vomiting, which again doesn't relieve. *Nux vomica* and *Arsenicum album* are mostly the two remedies needed for acute food poisoning. With both remedies you can feel very chilly and need to be covered.

Aloe is a good remedy for travelers' diarrhea. In this remedy there is a feeling of great insecurity, specifically in the bowels. It feels as if you could lose stool at any moment. When passing wind, you may pass stool so you always have to be at the toilet. There can be a lot of loud flatus with the stool and it is sputtering and/or hot. You can have a pain in the back with the stool. Emotionally, you can feel very insecure, being in unfamiliar places and feeling out of control of your situation.

Chamomilla is a great remedy for children's diarrhea. It looks like chopped eggs and spinach and has a rotten, offensive odor, like bad eggs. The diarrhea often comes with cramping colic and great peevishness. It is a remedy for diarrhea while teething.

Gelsemium is good when diarrhea is due totally to an anticipatory anxiety before an event of some sort.

See Chapter Five: Emotional Conditions, Anxiety section

COMBINATION STRATEGY If in doubt which remedy to give, mix one tablet of *Arsenicum album*, *Podophyllum* and *Veratrum album* together in two to four ounces of water and take one tsp. every one to three hours until change, depending on the severity of symptoms.

🖋 HERBAL CARE

Goldenseal tincture can be taken for most forms of diarrhea, especially by E coli infection but it should not to be taken in pregnant or breast feeding women, or taken for longer than two weeks. Ispaghula (named Fybogel or Isogel in the UK) or Isabgol or more commonly known as psyllium can be taken for both diarrhea and constipation. It originates from the plantago family and is used to bulk up food, aiding peristaltic action in constipation. In diarrhea it helps absorb liquid in the small intestine. It needs to be taken with enough water or it can have a choking effect as it becomes sticky very quickly. Medicinal charcoal can be taken for mild diarrhea (one tablespoon three times daily for two days). Ensure the charcoal is sterile through heating and the wood used is not poisonous.

Dysentery

Dysentery is a diarrhea mostly caused by amoebas or bacillus although initially it can be treated like any other type of diarrhea. Most diarrheas of travelers are not dysentery, but if symptoms don't clear up or get better after three days, it should be considered as it indicates that parasites or bacillus (Shigellosis) are involved. If it is amoebic dysentery, it can continue for a long time, beyond three weeks when more serious. In both situations there is often blood with the stool and much mucous and undigested food. With both amoebic and bacillary dysentery it is important to treat effectively, especially when traveling. It can lead to great depletion, weakness, dehydration, secondary liver problems (abscesses), eye problems, arthritis etc. It is useful to get a medical diagnosis of what type of dysentery it is. Both types are spread mostly through food and water, though flies can transmit the disease.

Bacillary dysentery may begin more suddenly in more serious cases, often with a fever (whereas amoebic dysentery often has no fever) and there can be severe cramping in the abdomen. Stools are very frequent, explosive, with much mucus, blood, watery and frothy diarrhea. It is often odorless. Cases may be mild and recover within a few days or may continue for up to three weeks. However, even when symptoms have disappeared, one can carry and spread the condition for some months.

Amoebic dysentery tends to start more slowly but then develops into more frequent copious stools than found in bacillary dysentery. Often one does not feel particularly unwell at this stage, in contrast to bacillary dysentery. It can be found both in temperate and tropical zones. Its severity is often dependent on the overall health of the person. Healthy people can catch this and have very mild symptoms which soon disappear. However, it can become a more chronic condition with intermittent symptoms of loose stool and also constipation which continues even for years. It will be aggravated by other factors such as diet, exhaustion and other diseases. If symptoms are more extreme and acute, the onset is sudden with frequent urging of offensive watery, mucus laden stools, which are very offensive. Stools may be involuntary, and there can be cramping and spasms in the rectum. In some cases, the amoebas reach the liver, with symptoms of fullness in the liver region (right upper quadrant of the abdomen, below the ribs), pain referred to the right shoulder, fever with sweating and loss of appetite and weight. Loss of weight and appetite can occur in any of the above situations.

In more serious cases, if symptoms do not get better within one week, then professional homeopathic care or other medical intervention should be sought.

● GENERAL CARE

Prevention is key through effective hygiene. Always wash your hands, especially after stool. Avoid bad food and water. Do not touch things unnecessarily. Be careful being around others as you can still spread the condition even when feeling better. Keep hydrated at all times. Do not eat food that aggravates the digestive system. Avoid spicy, creamy, rich foods and fruit. Keep the diet very minimal; plain rice, bananas, and other simple foods if the symptoms are severe. Yoghurt is OK as it helps replenish the bowel flora but it may not be digested too easily, so eat only small amounts. Conventional care involves appropriate antibiotics for bacillary dysentery and often Metronidazole (Flagyl) or Tinidazole for amoebic dysentery. Flagyl is also often given for giardia, but it can affect some people adversely and may not totally clear up the condition. It should be taken more as a last resort and natural methods tried first.

◆ HOMEOPATHIC CARE

China is the main remedy to consider, especially if there is great bloating and fullness in the abdomen. You can feel very exhausted, depleted and weak, which is much worse after stool. You have little appetite, feeling full after a few bites. Stool may be bloody and with mucus, and diarrhea may alternate with constipation. Passing gas doesn't relieve the bloating and the liver may also feel full and hard. It is often needed when the symptoms have become more chronic and long term. Initially diarrhea may be much worse after fruit and/or rich food. It is the main remedy for giardia.

Mercurius (vivus or solubulis) is one of the best remedies to take for more acute dysentery, (both amoebic and bacillary). There is frequent painful urging of bloody stool and there is very little relief after stool. The urging can be painful and fairly constant. Often the stool is very offensive, even metallic smelling and also perspiration can be offensive. You feel very 'toxic'. Fever is often present, but not too high. Perspiration is seen with fever, which can feel oily. There can be fullness in the liver region and great weakness and depletion. If there is much blood with the stool and a constant, ineffectual urging and unsatisfied feeling, then *Mercurius corrosivus* (another form of mercury) should be taken if *Mercurius* does not fully cure.

Baptisia is indicated in more serious states, when there is great exhaustion, depletion and achiness in the body. Stools are dark, thin, bloody and offensive. You can feel distension and rumbling and mentally you feel very low, confused, tired and tend to fall asleep very easily, even when being spoken to. Your face can look besotted and there is an ongoing low fever. *Arnica* can also be taken if it looks like *Baptisia* and it hasn't worked and there is soreness and aching in the body and the bed feels hard when lying down.

Sulphur is very useful in more chronic situations when the stool is very offensive, burning, bloody and with mucus. There may be great urging on waking in the morning. The rectum may burn intensely after stool and flatus can be very offensive. *Sulphur* should be given if you have tried other remedies which either haven't worked or only worked partially. All the remedies listed in the diarrhea section can also be thought of.

COMBINATION STRATEGY If no remedy is clear mix one tablet of *Baptisia*, *China* and *Mercurius* in two to four ounces of water and take one tsp. three to six times a day, depending on severity of symptoms.

HERBAL CARE

Take charcoal tablets and/or clay internally.

Food Poisoning

Food poisoning can happen at any time and in any place. It is often experienced traveling due to dirty food and water, yet it can occur equally when at home or eating at a restaurant. One of the most common causes is Salmonella bacteria and other bacteria and also some viruses. Symptoms tend to come on very suddenly and intensely and also often diminish within one to three days.

GENERAL CARE

If possible, keep fluid intake up but do not worry too much at the beginning. Endure the acute symptoms until you feel some improvement.

Do not eat anything until vomiting and acute diarrhea have decreased significantly.

Arsenicum album is the first remedy to take for simple food poisoning. There is sudden intense diarrhea and nausea and vomiting, which can all come on at the same time. Nausea is often worse at the sight or smell of food. *Veratrum album* has very similar symptoms but has more cold perspiration, especially on the forehead. Both have weakness and prostration after stool. *Nux vomica* is the next remedy to take, especially when there is great cramping in the abdomen and violent retching and vomiting, with the feeling that you just can't bring everything up. Spasms can be felt anywhere in the body and nausea is much worse from the smell of food. *Podophyllum* is useful when there is a lot of bloating, rumbling and gurgling in the intestines followed by a violent, forcible stool exploding from the rectum. There may also be cramping in the abdomen before stool.

Hemorrhoids

Hemorrhoids (piles) are due to enlarged varicose veins in the rectal area. They can come as a consequence of constipation, and some people are more predisposed to them than others. Recurrent pain and distress in the rectal area should be examined for its causation, as often such symptoms are simply put down to hemorrhoids when other factors may be at play. Piles may be internal or external or may be exposed only after straining at stool. Once piles have become chronic and seriously engorged, surgery can be required. However, homeopathic remedies can be very helpful in earlier stages. Constitutional treatment is usually the most effective approach to this condition.

● HOMEOPATHIC CARE

Nux vomica is the first remedy to consider for very sensitive, painful piles, especially due to overstraining when passing stool. The pain can be very intense and sharp and worse for any touch. *Aloe* also has piles from constipation which protrude and there is a great sense of pressure forcing downwards, creating insecurity in the region, as if stool can be lost, even if no diarrhea is there. There can be bleeding from the rectum and much wind. *Aesculus* is one of the main remedies for piles, with or without constipation. The main symptom is a sensation of sticks in the rectum and sharp pains extending up the back. There is a feeling of great congestion, fullness and burning in the rectum and the back can feel as if it is giving out. *Sulphur* is thought of if there is great heat and burning in the rectal area. If very sensitive piles are found along with cracks in the skin around the rectum, then *Nitric acid* can be given.

COMBINATION STRATEGY It may not be able to easily identify one remedy for this condition. If so, then mix one tablet of each remedy that seems indicated into four ounces of water and give one sip/tsp. three times daily for three days. Some relief should be seen by then.

Hepatitis

Hepatitis is an infection of the liver. There are three main types of hepatitis, termed A, B and C. Hepatitis A is the most common infection, occurring through contaminated water and is common in many developing countries. Hepatitis B and C are communicated through blood and symptoms can remain dormant for many years. In this case, we are only dealing with hepatitis A. There are two types of conventional prophylaxis for Hepatitis A, a human immunoglobulin injection and a vaccination. The former gives immunity for about four months while the latter will give a long lasting immunity. If you have previously had hepatitis A, you will normally have lifelong immunity to the disease. *See Chapter Sixteen: Prevention*

Symptoms of Hepatitis A develop between two and four weeks after initial infection and often begin with symptoms similar to the 'flu. There may be fever, general malaise and weakness, aching of the body, a slightly raised temperature and a great lack of appetite, often with nausea and vomiting. There may be a strong aversion to fatty food and alcohol. There may also be diarrhea and or constipation. More characteristic, if seen, is a tenderness in the right upper abdominal region (right quadrant), where the liver is found. The area may be tender to touch and to clothing as well as to any motion. Symptoms of jaundice may be seen in many but not all cases. When this occurs, the urine becomes dark yellow and the skin and eyes become yellow.

Acute symptoms last on average two to three weeks but if more serious or the person is already weak, then overall weakness and digestive problems can last much longer. However, most cases should resolve completely within two months. However, there can be relapses after this phase, especially if a person resorts to eating as before, increasing pressure on the liver. Appropriate medical care should be taken and the person needs to live a simple, relaxed lifestyle until full recovery has been made.

In cases of hepatitis with jaundice, other diseases such as malaria and yellow fever must also be considered.

Hepatitis B and C are transmissible through blood contamination, e.g., unprotected sex, sharing needles, even having dental treatment abroad or getting tattoos. Infection can remain dormant for up to 20-30 years. Around 20% of people will develop some symptoms and in a small percentage of cases, serious liver damage can occur. Initial symptoms can be similar to Hepatitis A and diagnosis is necessary to distinguish which type of Hepatitis it is. At other times, there is no acute phase of symptoms and more chronic liver problems are the first sign.

● GENERAL CARE

General rest is crucial. There may be much weakness, along with digestive issues, so it is imperative that the person is well looked after and ideally stays in one place. Clean water and clean simple food are important. No fats, rich food, meat, alcohol, drugs or any kind of stimulants should be taken for a minimum of two months. Fruit is OK, especially papaya if in the tropics. Full recovery may take longer than two months if serious and a simple diet will need to be sustained for quite some time.

◆ HOMEOPATHIC CARE

There are a number of remedies for hepatitis in its various stages and in the acute phase, remedies may be given for the fever and other symptoms. See Chapter Seven: Common Infections, Fever and Influenza. However, the following remedies are often indicated in acute hepatitis.

China is one of the main remedies for liver problems as well as for other digestive conditions. There is often great weakness along with abdominal bloating and a very low appetite. The least food fills you up, even a few mouthfuls, and bloats the stomach. Jaundice may or may not be there. You may have diarrhea or constipation and often much gas which doesn't give any relief. You may have fever, with great weakness and easy perspiration. There is often an aversion to fat, rich food and fruit can cause diarrhea. *Nux vomica* is needed when you have great irritability and weakness. You feel sensitive to all odors and noises and you can have great nausea with retching. This is made worse from eating or drinking and even the smell of food. There is often a great aversion to fatty, rich food and alcohol. There can be sensitivity in the liver area and initially often a great chill and coldness.

Chelidonium is one of the most important liver remedies in homeopathy. When you need this remedy, you often have a specific pain in the right upper quadrant of the abdomen, but which extends through the body to the back and/or up the back to lower right shoulder blade. You can have abdominal sensitivity and bloating and some increased irritability and weakness, especially in the afternoon. *Lycopodium* is very similar to *Chelidonium* and one of the great remedies for all liver problems. There is pain in the liver, often extending to the back, like *Chelidonium*, and with the pain there is great bloating of the abdomen, with much gas being passed. There is often an aversion to clothing around the waist. There can be great hunger but with fullness after a few mouthfuls, similar to *China*. There can be swelling of the liver. Symptoms can often feel worse between four to eight pm., and there is weakness and irritability on waking in the morning. *Lycopodium* is useful for chronic complications from hepatitis, even years after the initial infection. *Phosphorus* is often indicated when jaundice becomes more chronic and doesn't go away, or when jaundice is present without hepatitis infection. In acute hepatitis, *Phosphorus* is indicated if there is much craving for cold water, which is often vomited when it becomes warm in the stomach.

COMBINATION STRATEGY It is good to give a homeopathic remedy and also a herbal remedy to support the liver at the same time, even if it is the same remedy, one in a homeopathic dose, the other herbal. Also, one remedy may be needed in the beginning and then another remedy may follow as the picture changes. Pay attention to the symptom picture.

🌿 HERBAL CARE

Carduus mariannus (St. Mary's Thistle) tincture. Take as instructed for one to three weeks. This is both a homeopathic and herbal medicine, which can be taken to support the liver and spleen during hepatitis. It can be taken along with other homeopathic remedies.

Chelidonium (Greater Celandine) tincture can be taken in the same way as *Carduus mariannus* and is a good support for the liver. Milk thistle tincture is another excellent liver support remedy as is dandelion root.

Hiccough

Having a hiccough is a common enough condition, which seems to come on spontaneously. It may be related to how food and drink have been taken or by certain emotions and at times it can become a prolonged and debilitating condition. It is common in infants. In adults there are many solutions suggested, from drinking water upside down when bending down, breathing fast or slow or breathing into a paper bag etc.

🔻 HOMEOPATHIC CARE

Ignatia is the first remedy to consider when hiccoughs come from being disappointed or any other emotional cause. However, *Nux vomica* is more indicated if anger precipitated the hiccoughs and where they are particularly violent in nature. *Arsenicum album* may be good if the hiccoughs came on just after taking a cold drink or during a chill or fever.

Indigestion

This can be used as a catch-all phrase for upset stomach, including heartburn and can be caused by bad food, too much food and emotional anxiety. Many times, this is not a limited acute situation but reveals an underlying vulnerability in the digestive area. However, when there is any case of simple indigestion, it can be unpleasant and can lead to further problems, like Irritable Bowel Syndrome (IBS).

● GENERAL CARE

It is important to eat simple food if having any indigestion. Fatty, rich food, meat, fish and dairy products should be avoided. Acidic fruit and alcohol also should be avoided. Simple food should be taken. Papaya is excellent for indigestion. Ideally sap from a raw papaya can be taken, a few drops, mixed with some water.
See Chapter Seventeen: Homeopathic and Herbal Remedy list, Herbal and Plant remedies, Papaya section

● HOMEOPATHIC CARE

There are many remedies one can consider for this situation, which can also be found described in the diarrhea and dysentery sections. The most common of these is *Arsenicum album* which has the characteristic nausea, and vomiting and also diarrhea. If it is only a burning in the stomach along with just nausea, *Arsenicum album* is the first remedy to consider.

However, if bloating, tiredness, weakness and much eructation and gas are experienced, then *Carbo veg*etabalis and *China* should be considered. *Carbo veg*, which is made from vegetable charcoal, is excellent for simple indigestion, especially from eating too much rich food, fruit and ice cream. There is often weakness with distension of the abdomen. You may have lots of wind, with loud and at times rancid burps or much flatulence. All food seems to just turn to gas and clothing around the waist seems too tight. *China* has been well described in the dysentery and hepatitis sections.

Colocynthis and *Nux vomica* are two important remedies to consider especially when cramping pains are a key symptom. *Nux vomica* in particular is one of the most important remedies for indigestion that comes from simply eating too much food or too much rich, spicy food or too much alcohol. You can experience nausea and retching, a strong ineffectual urging to vomit and/or to pass stool. The stomach can feel very acidic with bitterness in the mouth and increased general irritability.

Colocynthis is described in the diarrhea section.

Pulsatilla is a good remedy for any effects of eating too much rich food, ice cream and bad fruit and where there is a feeling of a stone in the stomach after eating. There can be regurgitations tasting of food. *Sulphur* is needed if with indigestion, there are burning pains and eructations smelling or tasting like eggs. There can be great hunger, especially at 11am which comes with a sinking, weak feeling.

Nausea

There are many reasons why nausea occurs. Finding the correct homeo-pathic remedy depends on the reasons why the nausea is happening. Remedies are suggested partly according to the cause of the nausea and partly on the actual symptoms being experienced. The following conditions are common reasons for nausea and remedies will be found in the appropriate sections of the book: Anxiety, Cholera, Diarrhea, Fever, Food poisoning, Hangover, Indigestion, Kidney colic, Malaria, Poisonings, Pregnancy, Shock, Travel sickness, Typhoid etc.

◆ HOMEOPATHIC CARE

A few of the most important remedies for nausea, and when found indi-cated in many different conditions are *Arsenicum album*, *Cocculus*, *Ipecac*, *Nux vomica*, *Sepia*, *Tabacum* and *Veratrum album*. For basic descriptions of remedies for nausea, see Food Poisoning and Travel Sickness sections.

Worms

There are three main types of intestinal worms that one can catch while traveling or at home. Worm infections are very common in warmer climes and when hygiene is not so good and can affect very many people. In some people, there are little or no symptoms, while in others, symp-toms are stronger. Also the type of worm affects the type of symptoms. Conventional and homeopathic treatment may be undertaken to treat them.

Good hygiene and avoiding eating undercooked meat and unwashed uncooked vegetables are key factors in not getting worms.

1. Threadworms or Pinworms. These are the common type of worm often found in children. They are small thin worms, which are often found in the stool and the anus. They create great itching in the anus, especially at night and may also lead to itching in other parts of the body. It can lead to a general restlessness, irritability and loss of appetite and weight. In adults, it may be seen simply as an intense itching anus, worse at night. Worms may or may not be seen. Children often produce more symptoms, including mood changes, irritability and loss of appetite and weight.

2. Roundworms (Ascariasis). These are very common worms found in most parts of the world. Infection happens through ingesting eggs often found in raw vegetables. There may be no symptoms or signs of worms in the stool, anus or in vomit and in the nostrils. Some children, especially in developing countries may have serious infections, leading to malnutrition, with nausea, vomiting and diarrhea. Infection may even go to the liver, with symptoms of jaundice and may infect the lungs, with symptoms of cough, difficult respiration, fever etc.

3. Tapeworms. A tapeworm is a thin, long worm that can grow considerably in the intestine. It is often symptomless, or there may be some irritation in the anus region. Infection happens through eating raw or undercooked beef. Other types of tapeworms can be caught through eating raw or undercooked fish or in food contaminated with mouse droppings.

● **GENERAL CARE**

There are a number of ways to help purge worms from the system using natural methods. Some may work better than others. It is worth trying before using toxic drugs. Fasting or doing juice fasts for up to ten days can be effective, especially for pin worms. For round and tape worms, it is also important to purge the worms. Take one tablespoon of fresh coconut and then take about 50ml of castor oil mixed with around 300 ml of milk three hours later. (A non-dairy milk can be used). Repeat daily as needed. Or, take a teaspoon of powdered papaya seeds and mix with one cup of water and take daily on an empty stomach. Alternatively use Artemesia (wormwood) oil, mixing with olive oil (or coconut oil) in the ratio of 1 8-10. Take at least 50 ml of this and repeat daily. One can also use Artemesia oil in an enema form, using 2ml of oil in about 100ml of lukewarm water. Another option when in the tropics is to use the sap of an unripe papaya.

See Chapter Seventeen: Homeopathic and Herbal Remedy list, Herbal and Plant remedies, Papaya section

A natural laxative should be taken at the same time, e.g., ripe fruit like figs, mangoes or papaya. Mix with lots of water and ideally take in the morning or empty stomach.

◆ HOMEOPATHIC CARE

Cina is the first remedy for irritable children with worms. There is great itching of the anus and violent boring and picking of the nose. Mentally the child is very angry and capricious. Nothing satisfies and the child is ugly and petulant, throwing things away when given. There can be grinding of teeth at night. *Sabadilla* is good when there is great itching in the anus and skin and around the nose and ears. There is often itching in the palate of the mouth and twitching in many parts of the body. There is a watery, runny nose and eyes. *Teucrium marum verum* is needed for itching of the anus, worse at night with crawling and picking of the nose. The child is over excitable and sensitive and has difficulty to sleep.

Silicea is for children who have worms with itching and who are losing weight with no appetite. They become more reserved and timid and avoid company due to a lack of confidence. They become more chilly and have profuse, sour perspiration. *Sulphur* has great itching and burning in the anus and the skin in general, worse at night and when warm. There is offensive flatus and perspiration and the skin looks dirty. When no other remedy has relieved or only helped somewhat, *Sulphur* should be thought of.

NOTE Constitutional homeopathic care may be needed to fully resolve a worm infection. Sometimes homeopathic treatment is enough, either one of the remedies mentioned or a constitutional based remedy. However, conventional treatment can also be used. Fasting or doing a prolonged juice fast can be a good way of helping purge worms from the system (but not to be done by children or those already malnourished due to chronic worm infection).

🍃 HERBAL CARE

There are a number of ways to purge parasites. One is to take two tbs. of black walnut hull tincture, seven capsules of wormwood (See Artemesia above) and one capsule of cloves three times a day. Parsley tea can also be used.

Chapter Seven
Common Infections

Any common infection that involves a fever can be found here and influenza is included in this chapter as it is one of the most common conditions found. There are many reasons for fevers to occur, influenza being one of the most common, so identifying the key characteristics of remedies for both conditions is useful to know. Children's diseases are less likely to be seen today, but as they often come with a fever, they are included in this chapter.

Simple Fever

A fever is a natural body reaction to any type of infection. It is the way the body 'throws off' a disease through an increased level of activity of the body's immune system. It is important to find out why the fever is there. Which area is affected? Is there pain associated with the fever? It is good not to simply suppress a fever. There is a tendency to always want to do something. It is better to try and let the fever take its course or give the correct homeopathic remedy if the picture is clear.

Fevers are most often seen in children. Fevers up to 104f, (40 Celsius) are not unusual and if it comes down to around 100f (37.5 Celsius) fairly quickly after treatment, there is normally nothing to worry about. Fevers higher than 104f or which don't come down after treatment may require professional care. Any sign of a stiff neck, arching of the neck or pain in the area requires medical intervention as it may be meningitis.

Fevers occur in adults most often when having the 'flu, or when traveling due to a more serious tropical disease. Although the temperature may go as high as 104f (40 C), it is usually less than this. In most cases, do not suppress the fever with drugs. Take appropriate care and treatment and wait it out. Exceptions are when fever is associated with a potentially serious condition such as a kidney infection, blood poisoning, malaria or other serious infection in a part of the body. In these cases, there should be other symptoms to indicate the nature of the problem. *See Chapter Eight: Colds and Coughs, Chapter Nine: ENT, Chapter Eleven: Bladder and Kidney, Chapter Thirteen: Common Tropical Diseases*

● **GENERAL CARE**

Explore the possible causes of the fever – is there pain anywhere, swelling, or any other symptom? With viral cold infections, fever is often a generalized response to the virus and there is no specific area affected. With a fever, keep hydrated. Drink plenty of water. Do not get exposed to the cold. Keep warm, especially if the fever involves a chill. Eat only small amounts, if at all. If necessary, take a tepid bath or do a sponge bath with tepid water if the fever is exceptionally high. Cool the head down if there is heat. Do not let children get too hot with a fever but also refrain from using too many medications to suppress a fever unless it is very high. However, if the fever does not go down in a number of days or is getting exceptionally high, seek professional medical care.

● **HOMEOPATHIC CARE**

Many other remedies can have fever associated with them, but are not listed here. The remedies listed here are known for their fever symptoms alone, whereas with other remedies there will be other information to prescribe on. See the listed chapters above and also the Influenza section. It is important to check the area that may be infected, e.g., ear, bladder, throat etc., as there are other remedies that will be listed there which are more specific for those conditions. The remedies listed below are the main ones for a simple fever.

If the fever comes on very suddenly and intensely, then *Aconite* and *Belladonna* are often needed. *Aconite* has a high, often dry fever, with great thirst and much restlessness, anxiety and even anguish. Exposure to cold air may often be the cause of an *Aconite* type fever. There may an intense inflammatory process or disease, e.g., acute ear infection and much pain can be seen. Everything feels extreme and if it comes after an intense emotional shock, this confirms the remedy. *Belladonna* has a classic intense hot fever. You can feel as if burning up inside, the skin is hot and dry, the face flushed, the eyes staring and the pupils are dilated. It is often needed in children who suddenly spike a fever. There can be thirst for small sips or large amounts and even for lemonade. There can even be wild delirium with thrashing about and this is worse from any motion and jarring. It is the first remedy to consider for any sudden fever. *Apis* can also be given for fevers. Often it looks like *Belladonna* and there is often no thirst, even though very hot or the thirst comes when feeling chilled. If *Apis* is needed, it may indicate an infection of some other organ, e.g., kidney or bladder. Pains may be burning and stinging, and in the fever, the head is rolling from side to side. The skin will often be dark or bright red.

The fevers of *Bryonia*, *Eupatorium perfoliatum* and *Gelsemium* do not come on so suddenly or intensely. They develop more slowly but can also get quite high. In *Bryonia*, there is great dryness of the body and the mucous membranes, leading to a large thirst. There can also be delirium, at times saying "I want to go home", when already there. They often want to keep totally still, are worse from any jar and can be irritable and want to be left alone.

Eupatorium and *Gelsemium* are similar in that they both have extreme aching of the muscles and joints with the fever. That is why they are good 'flu remedies. Both remedies can have a strong chill, which goes up and down the back. *Eupatorium* often has more thirst than *Gelsemium* which can be thirstless. The pains in *Eupatorium* feel like their bones are breaking, most often felt in the back. There can also be nausea and vomiting with the fever, even of bile. Nausea is worse from the smell of food. *Gelsemium* has the intense aching of muscles and often feels sleepy, weak, dizzy and dull. The face can be besotted (confused and full looking), looking very dull and the eyelids feel too heavy to hold up, and even the head can feel too heavy to hold up.

Nux vomica is a great remedy for any fever associated with a 'stomach 'flu'. With the fever, there is great chill, wanting to be covered at all times and worse from any drafts, which is similar to *Arsenicum album* and *Rhus tox*. See Influenza below. You can feel much cramping in the stomach or back area and you can feel very irritable and very sensitive to any noise and smells. All senses are more acute. *Sulphur* is needed when there is burning and throbbing of any part of the body with the fever and you feel indifferent and disconnected to what is going on around you. It is good when there doesn't seem a clear picture for any other remedy but something is definitely going on.

🌿 HERBAL CARE

Make a tea with a combination of elderflower, yarrow and peppermint. Also boneset tea can be used. Using eucalyptus and tea tree oil in fevers and 'flu can be useful, adding it to some steaming water for a vapor effect. Elderberry juice has been used for generations against fever, influenza and other viral and bacterial conditions. Lemon grass tea is good to take for any fever, one to two liters per day.

Influenza

We often say we have the 'flu when we simply have a bad cold. True influenza is due to particular viruses and historically we have been getting forms of the 'flu for thousands of years. Spread from animals such as birds and pigs, they have contaminated humans and led to outbreaks of influenza.

There are various strains of influenza, creating the challenge to find a vaccine for the current strain, which changes each year. They are classified according to their make-up, and given titles such as HIN1, H5N1 etc. This relates to the genetic code of the virus. However, whatever type of 'flu it is, they are relatively mild for most people and can be treated effectively with homeopathy. A healthy constitution generally helps mitigate more serious complications of most 'flus. The most serious and frequent complication of the 'flu is pneumonia, which occurs mainly in children under two and in seniors. The viral form of pneumonia can be very serious and requires instant treatment. It comes on very quickly whereas bacterial pneumonia is slower to develop. .

The fear today is of a new strain of 'flu virus arriving that we have no genetic immunity to, contaminating humans through connections with certain animals and then mutating into a virulent form of the virus, similar to the 1918 'Spanish 'flu' epidemic, in which up to 30 million people died. In the normal course of affairs, once someone has had the 'flu, immunity is developed to the same strain and even to slightly different strains. The concern is when a totally different strain is seen which would affect healthy young people as much as the elderly and infants.

The effectiveness of influenza vaccines being offered varies from year to year and the overall effectiveness is disputable. In the elderly, the original focus for the vaccine, the lack of effectiveness can be due to their diminishing immune response due to age. According to the Centers for Disease Control (CDC), the effectiveness of the 'flu vaccine among elderly in nursing homes is 30-40%. It may be even lower than that. Also, the 'flu vaccines do have significant side effects.

Due to the increased concern of a new virulent form of influenza, it is important to ensure that you take all precautions against the 'flu and also to treat any symptoms effectively. Anti viral treatments may work against some 'flu viruses but there are no guarantees. The effect of Tamiflu, for example, is already very limited in many cases of 'flu infection.
See Chapter Sixteen: Prevention, Influenza

● **GENERAL CARE**

It is important to rest when signs of the 'flu are there and to keep hydrated. Do not get overexposed to the cold and keep warm.

◗ **HOMEOPATHIC CARE**

The remedies mentioned are similar for many other types of viral and bacterial infections. The most important thing is to identify the main characteristics of each remedy, irrespective of the name of the condition. Remedies have been separated according to certain stages of the 'flu which are often seen.
See Chapter Eight: Cold and Coughs

1st stage of symptoms when high fever predominates.

All remedies in the Fever section can be considered here. However, in the first stages when symptoms develop, if it is an intense and sudden onset of symptoms with fever, then *Aconite* and *Belladonna* are the most common remedies. The intensity of heat, high fever, thirst and throbbing congestion of blood, especially in the head are important symptoms. *Aconite* is more restless, anxious and fearful and the thirst is stronger. In *Belladonna* there can be more wildness and delirium with the fever, often with dilated pupils, a red complexion and a wild look in the face.

Bryonia also has heat and a bad headache, like *Belladonna* but the symptoms develop more slowly and they are more irritable, desire to be left alone and also like *Belladonna* don't want to be moved at all. They can have delirium as well, but it is more passive.

Arsenicum album has fever and heat alternating with chill and extreme restlessness and anxiety. *Rhus tox* also has great restlessness and also heat alternating with chill. The chill is worse for any uncovering and the restlessness is less to do with anxiety and more simply a need to move around. Both can be restless during fever and especially at night in bed. *Rhus tox* also has a strange symptom of redness on the tip of the tongue, while *Arsenicum album* may have a white coated tongue, like paint.

1st stage with fever but body aching predominates. (Also include remedies above)

Gelsemium is the most commonly prescribed remedy for 'flu when aching of the body predominates. The aching is felt in the muscles all over the body, but especially the back. There is fever and chills, which are felt especially going up and down the back. Often with fever, there is no thirst. The strongest symptoms are aching, with drowsiness, dullness and a weak feeling. Even the eyelids seem too heavy to hold open. *Eupatorium perfoliatum* can often look like *Gelsemium*. However the aching is felt more in the bones, as if they are breaking. It is a deep ache and often felt in the back. There is also fever and chill, and like *Gelsemium*, it goes up and down the back. There can be intense shaking with the chill and also nausea and vomiting, even of bile. *Bryonia* and *Rhus tox* can also have intense aching and are described above.

When there is great soreness and a bruised feeling with aching, with great exhaustion and an ongoing state of low fever in protracted 'flu, then remedies like *Arnica* and *Baptisia* can be given. In *Arnica* you feel sore and don't want to be touched or even approached. You can toss and turn and feel as if the bed is too hard. That feeling of the bed being too hard is common to both remedies. In *Baptisia*, the main sensation is a great weakness, drowsiness and feeling extremely languid. It is like *Gelsemium* but even more weak and prostrated. In a fever state, you can feel as if parts of your body are scattered about the bed. There can be a foul odor of the body and a septic feeling in the body. There may be diarrhea/dysentery with 'flu symptoms.

2nd stage when weakness, exhaustion and depletion predominate.

For symptom pictures, see above. This weak state may come on quickly in a 'flu state or may develop more slowly as the condition gets worse and you feel as if you are sinking deeper into the condition. If the weakness does come on quickly, then remedies like *Arsenicum album* and *Rhus tox* can be thought of. If symptoms develop more slowly, then *Gelsemium* is often the remedy. However in more serious states with great weakness and prostration, then *Arnica*, *Baptisia* and also *Pyrogen* can be thought of. This last remedy looks like *Baptisia*, has great soreness and also low fever with offensive discharges and odor. It feels septic and is useful for any fever that comes from a septic infection. One symptom is that the pulse can either be much too quick or too slow for the condition. It is often indicated in serious conditions like typhoid, malaria or pelvic infections.

3rd stage when lung symptoms predominate, including hemorrhage and pneumonia

This is a very serious stage of the 'flu and can be caused by other infections. Appropriate medical care should be sought. Homeopathy can be used alongside conventional treatment. Check for remedy information in Fever section and in Chapter Eight: Colds and Coughs.

COMBINATION STRATEGY You can combine one or more remedies that seem similar to the symptoms being seen. It is not always easy to find the exact remedy but look for the most important characteristics to help make a decision. Mix one tablet of the remedies chosen into a glass of water, and take one tsp. every one to four hours, depending on the severity of symptoms. Some change should be seen between 12-24 hours but it may take a couple of days to feel real improvement.

NOTE Professional homeopathic and other medical care should be sought to address serious conditions and also for any consequences after the 'flu. Some people find it very difficult to recover after serious 'flu and their immune systems remain low for a period of time. Homeopathy can be effective in addressing this situation.

🌿 HERBAL CARE

Echinacea tincture 30 drops hourly or three to four times a day depending on severity of symptoms. It can also be taken to prevent the 'flu and can be taken in a homeopathic dose for ailments that have stemmed from the 'flu. As mentioned for fever, eucalyptus and tea tree oil can be used in hot water. Elderberry juice can be taken as well. Ginger and cinnamon tea can be taken.

Taking larger doses of Vitamin C are often taken to help prevent and address 'flu symptoms. Vitamin D3 can be taken during the 'flu season as prevention.

See Chapter Sixteen: Prevention

Common Children's Diseases.

The following diseases used to be very common for nearly all children to get when fairly young. If the child was healthy they would be relatively mild and the vast majority would get better within a few days to one week. However, most children in the developed, and now the developing world, are vaccinated against these diseases and the incidence of them has declined in early childhood. However, homeopaths and other natural health practitioners believe that having some of these diseases serves a purpose in stimulating the body's natural immune system and also after having had these diseases, one has a lifelong immunity. That is not the case with vaccines. There is evidence of the vaccine wearing off, leaving children and adults potentially exposed to the diseases at a later stage of life when they can be much more serious. Also, we have developed a genetic immunity to the more serious expressions of these diseases, which has been passed on through generations. This is now not happening due to the vaccines being used, and children of vaccinated parents will not have the same immunity as a child of a parent who had the diseases. Cultures who did not have any genetic immunity to these diseases tended to get them much more severely, leading to many deaths, e.g., when Captain Cook arrived in Hawaii and other Pacific islands he inadvertently brought with him the diseases of his culture that devastated both indigenous children and adults who had no natural immunity. This was the same throughout the world when colonists and travelers came across various indigenous cultures. Therefore, there is a case to be made that having the diseases offers greater immunity for life and also that using 'live' vaccines, where the material used is still live may lead to a genetic mutation of the disease over time.

When traveling abroad with children who have been vaccinated, there is a small chance that the vaccine will not give full immunity if the child (or adult) is exposed to the disease, especially in developing countries, where it may be more commonly experienced. However, the chances are fairly small and vaccines for these diseases are not normally offered for basic travel.

With all the following conditions, there may be fever. If so, the child should be kept warm and comfortable. Avoid suppressing the fever unless it is very high but keep the child well hydrated and fed simple food as needed.

Chicken Pox

This is a common childhood illness, which is not seen as much today because of vaccinations. It is mostly a benign disease when acquired as a child, but can be much more serious when caught as an adult. One study revealed that children vaccinated more than three years previously were at a greater risk of the disease than those vaccinated more recently. It is a highly infectious disease so the infected person should be kept away from other people. However, most unvaccinated children are not likely to get the disease now as its incidence has declined due to vaccination.

The incubation period is about two weeks after the primary infection and when skin eruptions appear.

See Chapter Twelve: Skin Conditions, Shingles section

NOTE   It is possible that the vaccine, using a live virus may implant the varicella zoster virus into the cells of the nervous system, leading to shingles at a later stage of life.

● GENERAL CARE

All the eruptions should be kept clean and covered with band aids or clothing. *Calendula* cream can be used to protect the open sore. Oatmeal baths can be used to help the itching.

◆ HOMEOPATHIC CARE

The first remedy to consider is *Rhus tox*. There is great itching with the vesicles and often restlessness and anxiety. *Pulsatilla* is another remedy to consider when the emotional symptoms predominate, with weepiness, complaining and a need for consolation. This will obviously be seen more in children and if there is a fever, little thirst will be seen. *Sulphur* can be given when there is great itching and burning of the skin, which is worse from warmth. *Sulphur* can also be used if the other remedies are tried but don't finish the job.

See Chapter Seven: Common Infections, Fever and Influenza

⬤ HERBAL CARE

Tea tree oil or lavender can be used to soothe any eruption sores, as with the other children's conditions. Neem oil can also be used.

German Measles

German measles is a viral disease that also used to be very common in children before widespread vaccination. For young children, the symptoms are generally very mild and often disappear after a few days. For older people, there may be secondary joint pains and in pregnant women there can be birth defects if caught in the first trimester.

HOMEOPATHIC CARE

Aconite is needed if symptoms come on very suddenly with high fever and restlessness. *Belladonna* is needed when symptoms begin suddenly, with the characteristic burning heat, throbbing head, dilated pupils with a wild look in the face. *Pulsatilla* is needed if the child is weepy, clingy and complaining and also has yellow/green discharge and a loose cough.

Measles

Measles is not seen that much in the developed world now, but children may get it if exposed when traveling. Also, vaccinated children may get it later in life if exposed to the virus as the vaccine does not necessarily confer lifelong immunity. Adults are now being recommended, at least in the United States, to have booster doses one to two times before 60 years old.

HOMEOPATHIC CARE

If your child has been exposed to someone with measles, you can immediately give *Pulsatilla* three times a day for two days as a preventative measure. It may lessen the attack if infected. At the first stages of the condition, *Aconite* and *Belladonna* may be needed. *Bryonia* is also an excellent remedy for measles especially when there is irritability and wanting to be alone during the fever. *Euphrasia* is useful when there are very strong eye symptoms involved with inflammation, lachrymation (watering of eyes) and conjunctivitis, and *Pulsatilla* when the child is very weepy and clingy. *Sulphur* is needed when the skin symptoms are strongest, with great itching, which is much worse in the heat.

Mumps

Another of the 'children's diseases' rarely seen now, it was usually a mild infection when caught as a child. However, adult infection can lead to complications, especially inflammation of the testicles, which can lead to infertility. Mumps is normally seen with an inflammation and swelling of the parotid gland found on the side of the face in front of the ear.

Aconite or *Belladonna* may be needed initially. *Rhus tox* is another major remedy for mumps, when there is stiffness of the neck with swelling of the parotids and the neck and submaxillary glands. *Pulsatilla* is also indicated if the child is particularly weepy and clingy and both *Rhus tox* and *Pulsatilla* are good when the testicles are inflamed along with other symptoms.

Whooping Cough

Whereas there is an argument that diseases such as measles, chicken pox, mumps and german measles are 'natural' diseases that serve to stimulate a child's immune system, whooping cough does not necessarily fit into the same category and should be avoided at all costs.

Whooping cough is also known as Pertussis and is a bacterial infection that commonly affects young children. The most dangerous time to catch whooping cough is in the first year of life (especially the first six months) when the disease can be fatal, due to secondary pneumonia infection or convulsions due to the intensity of the cough. The most characteristic thing about whooping cough is the nature of the cough, in which a high pitch whooping noise can sometimes be heard as the child catches his/her breath after intense coughing. The difficulty in breathing is the most stressful thing about the cough and often it can be associated with a fever. The disease may last a number of weeks. Conventional treatment is mostly with antibiotics and cough suppressants.

A vaccine has been available since the 1940's but its effectiveness and safety has been widely disputed for many years. As the vaccine is normally first given at two months of age, it is a particularly susceptible time in a child's development and many acute and chronic consequences have been seen with the vaccine, including encephalitis, meningitis, learning disorders, Autism Spectrum Disorder etc. By the 1990's, a new 'acellular' vaccine replaced the 'whole-cell' vaccine, on grounds of improved safety, although this has been disputed.

There are new outbreaks of whooping cough among children in various countries, the majority of them having been vaccinated. Some children under the age of two months (the time when the first vaccine is given) have caught the disease, at times with fatal consequences. Also, vaccinated children can often get whooping cough but the symptoms are not characteristic of the classic whooping cough – the vaccine creating a distorted form of the cough - and therefore it is not always diagnosed as being whooping cough.

Adults, while traveling, are unlikely to come across whooping cough but it is possible that being around children a lot could increase the possibility of getting the disease. Most children, even in developing countries, are vaccinated now, so in theory, they should not be any more likely to catch the disease while traveling than at home. Children, if traveling, could possibly get the disease, especially if spending much time with other children, but it is not a disease to worry about while traveling any more than at home. However, if traveling with a child and he/she has a serious cough which doesn't go away, it is important to get professional medical care.

● HOMEOPATHIC CARE

The most important and first remedy to consider for whooping cough is *Drosera*. The cough is hard, barking, loud and often worse in the evening and night, especially when the child first lies down. There can be retching and vomiting with the cough, with violent paroxysm of cough following one another. *Cuprum* is another remedy to consider when there are great spasms in the throat (larynx/trachea) area while coughing and bringing up phlegm, and the child's face turns blue from the cough with a great feeling of suffocation. Swallowing water can relieve the cough. *Ipecac* is also an important remedy, with gagging and vomiting with the cough. Also there can be nosebleeds with the cough and the face also turns blue and there is a suffocative feeling.

See Chapter Eight: Colds and Coughs

COMBINATION STRATEGY If you cannot choose one remedy in the case of whooping cough, put one tablet of *Drosera*, *Cuprum* and *Ipecac* into two to four ounces of water, stir well and give one tsp. of liquid every five to ten minutes if the cough is extreme and every fifteen minutes if less so and keep giving it until some relief is seen. If that doesn't work, check for another remedy in the cough section. Get professional attention if serious, especially in very young babies.

Chapter Eight

Colds And Coughs

Colds

A cold is the generic term given for an infection, usually viral, which affects the eyes, nose and throat. It can lead to secondary infections of the sinuses, larynx/trachea and lungs. When traveling, 'new' viruses tend to afflict people with unusual colds. There may be a general fever but also it can be localized in the head region with no fever. If there is a cough with the cold, look at the Cough section for more remedy descriptions and Chapter Seven: Common Infections, and Chapter Nine: ENT.

● **GENERAL CARE**

Rest as much as possible. Do not take long trips or expose yourself to the cold and general elements. Drink plenty of fluids, both cold and hot, and eat well. If the nose is very congested, use steam to help open up the breathing passageways.

◆ **HOMEOPATHIC CARE**

It is good to pay attention to the type of weather if you catch a cold as it can help in finding a remedy. In cold, dry weather or when exposed to a cold wind and symptoms come on suddenly, with perhaps a fever, heat and chill, then *Aconite* is the most likely remedy. You may have all the normal symptoms of a runny nose etc., but the key symptoms are the suddenness of the symptoms, with a burning fever, intense thirst and mentally you may feel restless and anxious. *Arsenicum album* can look very similar but often the discharge from the eyes and nose is more burning and acrid, the symptoms don't come on so quickly and intensely but you tend to be chilly and restless, often more chilly than *Aconite*. The key is the focus on the eyes and nose, along with chilliness and restlessness. *Nux vomica* also looks like *Arsenicum album*, but has more intense sneezing and less burning of the eyes and nose. There can be great irritability with symptoms and feelings of great chill with shaking, which becomes worse when drinking cold drinks.

Allium cepa is the classic remedy for a cold when all the symptoms revolve around the eyes, nose and throat, with great watering of the eyes and nose and great irritation and burning in the eyes. There can be a tickling cough coming from the larynx, with a tearing pain when coughing, which is often worse in a warm room. *Sabadilla* is very similar to *Allium cepa*, but has more violent sneezing and also itching of the upper mouth (palate).
See Chapter Nine: ENT, Allergies

🌿 HERBAL CARE

Take echinacea and/or goldenseal tincture ten drops hourly for one day. Also take ginger tea. Take the echinacea for up to ten days. It is most effective when taken at the beginning of a cold. Eucalyptus oil can be used as an inhaler, with some drops put into hot water and steamed.

Coughs
including bronchitis and pneumonia

Coughs occur for many reasons and it is important to know the reasons for the cough, whether it is just a mild, self-limiting condition or indicative of something more serious, e.g., pneumonia. Often, it is associated with some of kind of bacterial or viral infection. The following are the most obvious remedies for many coughs, including whooping cough, which is also discussed in Chapter Seven. If whooping cough is seen in a small child, it is important to have professional medical care available.

It is useful to look at all sections in Chapter Seven for more remedies as coughs are often part of a cold and/or influenza and also Chapter Nine: ENT. It is not always easy to find the right homeopathic remedy for a cough. It is very important to find out what features make the cough worse or better, e.g., warm or cold weather, food or drink, talking, lying down, sitting up, etc. Also, pay attention to what the cough sounds and feels like, e.g., hacking, dry, wet, racking, barking etc. All this helps in choosing the correct remedy. You are becoming a homeopath!

Bronchitis is a bacterial infection in the bronchioles of the lung, leading at times to a fever, intense cough, exhaustion and general depletion. It may occur after a more superficial cold has gone 'deeper' into the lungs. It can become a chronic condition or can frequently recur in people sensitive to the condition. Often it is experienced as an intense cough that does not seem to go away by itself. It may or may not be associated with a fever. Remedies suggested include those for pneumonia, a deeper infection of the lungs than bronchitis. This can require medical intervention, especially in elderly people and when as a complication of influenza or other general infections.

● **GENERAL CARE**

Ensure enough water is taken for hydration. Keep warm. Do not move too much or aggravate the cough by violent exertion. Try and allow the mucus to come up, if there is some. Warm drinks may help loosen mucus. Use lozenges if necessary. If the cough is dry and irritating and especially worse at night, mix some honey, cider vinegar and a pinch of cayenne pepper together in a small amount of hot water and sip as needed. Other natural methods may work as well.

It is very distressing when children experience a sudden, intense cough. Croup (a cough with a spasm in the larynx causing breathing to be impeded) can be very intense as it seems the child is suffocating. Then suddenly the child will breathe in deeply making a strange sound and is then relieved for a bit. It is important to sit the child up. Attacks happen mostly at night and in children older than two years. The cough itself is hard, barking, violent and the cough seems to be suffocating the child. It is important to know if this is just a case of croup or whether the suffocative breathing is due to any other factor, including something stuck in the air passage. Whooping cough is also very similar to this and the same remedies are indicated although whooping cough is most serious in infants. There is also a condition where the epiglottis is swollen at the back of the tongue and this may be interfering with breathing. Immediate medical care should be sought. *Aconite* should be given to help matters while waiting for medical care.

● HOMEOPATHIC CARE

The most important factors in choosing which remedy you need are the sound of the cough and what makes it better or worse. This is the same whether we are looking at whooping cough, croup, bronchitis, pneumonia or just a simple cough. However, knowing the type and depth of infection can be important in helping identifying the remedy and also when a more serious infection is taking place.

When you have a cough that is hard, barking, choking, or like a croup, then *Aconite*, *Drosera* and *Hepar sulph* are important remedies. In *Aconite*, the cough may come on very quickly and is often worse at night. Any cough with intense fear and anxiety indicates *Aconite*. *Drosera* is one of the best remedies for many types of cough, especially when it is barking and hard. It is the first remedy to think of for whooping cough. There can even be retching and vomiting with the cough and it is often worse at night as soon as you put your head on the pillow. In *Hepar sulph*, the cough sounds similar but it is much worse from any cold air and better from warm drinks. You may even hear a rattle in the chest with great choking. *Spongia* is another remedy that has a very characteristic barking cough, which is like a seal bark or a saw going through wood. It is excellent for whooping cough and croup and when there is great dryness in the larynx/trachea area. The cough is better from drinking cold water.

Bryonia has one of the most painful of coughs and either the head, throat and chest needs to be held while coughing, similar to *Drosera* and *Phosphorus*. The cough of *Drosera* can sound similar. Any movement makes it worse and the cough is mostly dry, hard and hacking and is often worse in a warm room. *Belladonna* is similar to *Bryonia* with a dry, intense, painful and barking cough and both can have fever with the cough. They are important remedies in the first stages of bronchitis, especially when fever comes with the cough. There can be a great desire to drink due to dryness in the mouth and throat.

You may need *Arsenicum album* when, along with the cough there is a great burning feeling in the chest and also much restlessness and anxiety. Burning may also be felt in all the mucus membranes and the cough is mostly dry and hacking and often worse around midnight.

Ipecac and *Pulsatilla* have a much looser, more rattling type of cough. In *Ipecac*, the rattling cough often comes with nausea, retching and vomiting, the face turning red when coughing. You can feel as if you are suffocating with the cough and it is needed in croup, whooping cough, bronchitis and pneumonia. With the rattling in the chest, it can be hard to bring mucus up. In croup and whooping cough it is similar to *Drosera*. *Coccus cacti* is also similar, with production of much stringy, sticky mucus with the cough and/ or has intense vomiting along with the mucus. The cough is intensely tickling and violent, with a red face with the cough. In *Pulsatilla*, the cough is often associated with other conditions, such as conjunctivitis, sinusitis, otitis media or bronchitis. It is mostly loose and mucus from the chest or nose is yellow and/or yellow/ green. It is much worse in a warm room and better in the open air and is also much worse from lying down. *Pulsatilla* is a great children's remedy for coughs and colds.

In *Phosphorus*, the cough is usually dry and hacking and often there is tightness in the chest and a feeling of emptiness in the chest. The cough is often worse from a change in temperature, going from warm to cold or vice versa. It is one of the most important remedies in bronchitis and pneumonia and when intense the cough can rack the whole body. The person suffering often feels weak and exhausted.

If bronchitis has moved to becoming pneumonia and you are feeling very exhausted and seem unable to recover, then a few other remedies are useful. *Antimonium tart* is excellent for pneumonia when you feel as if you are drowning in mucus and can't get enough breath. The cough is deep, loose and suffocating, along with great rattling and wheezing. It is very hard to bring up mucus and it is exhausting trying to do so, making you feel pale and sweaty. It feels as if your lungs are becoming paralyzed. *Carbo vegetabilis* is another remedy when you feel as if you are really struggling with the cough. You feel totally exhausted, sweaty and cold and feel as if you can't get enough oxygen. You may want to be fanned, even though you are cold. Your face may turn blue and you can feel burning and rattling in the lungs. *Lachesis* is a similar state, with blueness of the face and where there is blood in the sputum being coughed up. The breathing is characteristically much worse on falling asleep and on waking.

If some of these remedies have been given and only worked partially and it is hard to get back to normal, then you should give *Sulphur* three times a day for three days. There may be residual burning in the lungs, weakness and the cough often wakes you at night.

COMBINATION STRATEGY If you are unsure of which remedy and the cough is croupy, choking and/or barking in nature, combine one tablet of *Aconite*, *Drosera* and *Hepar sulph* in water and take two to four times a day, depending on the intensity of the cough. If that doesn't work give *Spongia*. If it is pneumonia, with great weakness and a loose, rattling cough, which makes the person feel as if suffocating, you can combine *Antimonium tart*, *Carbo veg* and *Ipecac* and take as described above.

🍃 HERBAL CARE

Eucalyptus oil can be inhaled with bronchitis and with general colds. Do not inhale at the same time as taking a homeopathic remedy.

Chapter Nine
ENT: Ears, (Eyes, Mouth) Nose And Throat

Allergies

Allergies are mostly due to a reaction of the body to external factors (pollen, trees, dust, animals, feathers, etc.), which creates a histamine reaction in the body, leading to a variety of symptoms mainly affecting the eyes, nose, throat, chest, and skin. Hayfever is an allergy that often occurs at particular times of the year. Contact dermatitis is an allergy to certain irritants exposed onto the skin. If an allergy looks like it is becoming serious and is affecting the respiration and or the throat, or it is known that a serious reaction can happen, for example, from a bee sting, immediate medical attention should be sought.

Food allergies are not discussed here in particular and normally require more constitutional treatment. However, in more acute situations, remedies can be given.

See Chapter Six: Digestive Conditions. Also see the Conjunctivitis section and Chapter Eight: Colds and Coughs

🔴 HOMEOPATHIC CARE

Allergies can be treated two ways with homeopathy:
- Simply treating the acute symptoms while they are happening.
- Treating the underlying cause of the allergies, with

'constitutional' care. The focus here is on treating the acute symptoms.

One of the main remedies for simple allergies is *Allium cepa*. The focus is on the streaming eyes, which can burn and also profuse nasal discharge. There can be a tearing cough coming from the laryngeal area, feeling as if the throat is being torn apart. Two other similar remedies when the eyes and nose symptoms predominate are *Euphrasia* and *Sabadilla*. *Euphrasia* can also be taken in an eyedropper form. It has burning from the eyes and much streaming and often has inflammation of the conjunctiva of the eye. *Sabadilla* treats similar eye and nose symptoms, but also profuse intense sneezing and there may be itching in the upper palate of the mouth. *Nux vomica* is good when you feel extreme irritability with allergies and there is violent sneezing and *Arsenicum album* if you have much anxiety and restlessness, with burning of eyes, mouth, nose or skin.

In hayfever and general allergies, when the nose is obstructed with acrid discharge and sneezing, with a great desire to pick and bore at the nose, then *Arum triphyllum* is useful. There is great rawness in the mouth and throat and hawking from the throat and a hoarse voice. *Dulcamara* is good for hayfever when symptoms are much worse after damp weather or when exposed to a damp climate or house, especially after having been heated and then suddenly chilled.

If allergies are on the skin, then think of *Urtica urens*, *Rhus tox*, and *Apis*. *Apis* is the first remedy to think of for serious systemic allergy when the respiration is affected and threatens to close up the throat. There may be intense, burning, stinging and puffiness on the skin, especially around the eyes and there can be heat and a craving for open air. This is the remedy for threatened anaphylaxis when you may need immediate medical intervention. Give *Apis* in a 200c potency ideally, in water every one minute and get medical attention. *Urtica urens* is a good remedy for food allergies with hives which burn and itch. A shellfish allergy in particular indicates this remedy. *Rhus tox* is good for skin symptoms with many blisters (vesicles) and for intense burning, itching and restlessness.

Remedies can be taken one to five times a day depending on severity of symptoms. If more than twice a day, take the remedy in water and take one tsp. for each dose.

See Chapter Twelve: Skin Conditions, Poison oak

COMBINATION STRATEGY If you cannot find one remedy to match the symptoms you are feeling, then put one tablet of each indicated remedy into two to four ounces of water and take one sip three to five times daily for two to three days or until relief.

Cold Sores (Herpes)

These are herpetic eruptions on the lips, mostly experienced as a lumpy swelling, which can be red and irritating. There may be blistering of the area, with pustules/vesicles. Often these are chronic conditions which come out in times of stress but can also come from exposure to sun, dehydration, other current infections and also for no apparent reason. These are different to canker sores which are ulcerations of the lip and mouth. For some people, this is more of a chronic condition and therefore requires more constitutional treatment.

If you have an outbreak of cold sores, do not go into the sun; keep the area moist with lip cream.

● HOMEOPATHIC CARE

If you have an intense outbreak take *Rhus tox* when the lips burn and itch intensely, often with vesicles and where there is an achy feeling in the body. If cold sores appear especially on the center of the lower lip and are worse from exposure to the sun or come after an emotional upset, take *Natrum muriaticum*, one tablet three times daily for two days.

❧ HERBAL CARE

Take L-Lysine topically and internally. Goldenseal and tea tree, lavender and peppermint oil can be applied to the sore.

Ear Pain

Ear pain is often a result of an accumulation of mucus behind the ear drum, creating pressure and pain. There may a bacterial infection involved or it may be a consequence of a general viral infection which may lead to a secondary bacterial infection. An inner ear infection is called otitis media. Antibiotics are commonly given, especially for children, but often there is no bacterial infection so they do not work in those cases. Pain may also be caused by inflammation in the outer canal of the ear that leads to the eardrum. This is more easily treatable and less serious than an inner ear infection and is due to bacterial or fungal infection, often because of a tropical climate and hygiene challenges.

● GENERAL CARE

If there is a general fever, do not routinely give anti-inflammatory medicines, (tylenol etc.). A fever is a natural reaction of the body. It should only be suppressed if the fever is very high, or the person (especially a child) is in severe discomfort. It is hard to watch a child suffer so using homeopathic remedies along with anti-inflammatory medicines is OK. Treat the fever by keeping the person cool, using a cool wash cloth and even taking a tepid bath. Keep the person hydrated. Drinking water is extremely important. When lying down, lie on the opposite side to the ear pain. For external ear infections clean well, using *Calendula* or *Hypericum* tincture in warm water. Be careful not to push anything too far into the ear such as cotton plugs etc.

See Chapter Seven: Common Infections, Fever, Influenza

◆ HOMEOPATHIC CARE

There are many remedies for acute ear pain/infection. When there is a sudden attack of ear pain, the pain comes suddenly and is often associated with a fever, then *Aconite* and *Belladonna* are often needed. *Aconite* is the first remedy when symptoms come on after exposure to a cold wind and then suddenly there is great pain in the ear and a high fever. Use *Belladonna* for a bursting, throbbing pain in the ear and the fever is mostly dry, burning and with a red face and/or ear.

Hepar sulph and *Mercurius* are needed when there is an infection with the accumulation of pus behind the ear. The fever is not so high as *Aconite* or *Belladonna*, but both remedies have a sharp, stitching pain in the ear and the pain is worse from swallowing. In *Hepar sulph* it feels like a splinter in the ear. The pain often moves from the ear to the throat and back and the pain is much worse from any swallowing and you feel very chilly in general. The ear pain is better from warm applications and worse from any cold. You may feel very touchy and angry and there can be offensive discharge from the ear. *Mercurius* is one of the great ear, nose and throat remedies, and often ear problems are connected to throat infections. There is often offensive breath and a metallic taste, with increased saliva-tion, especially at night. There can be a low fever, often alternating with a chill, with shaking and trembling and offensive perspiration. *Mercurius* can often be given after *Hepar sulph* if it has not finished the job.

Two other remedies to consider are *Chamomilla* and *Pulsatilla*. *Chamomilla* is known as the remedy for pain. When you need *Chamomilla*, you can feel as if the pain is unendurable. Nothing seems to relieve it. It is one of the first remedies to give to children with ear pains. Mentally, the child can be angry, capricious and does not want to be touched or disturbed. The child often shrieks with the pain. The same applies if seen in an adult. In *Pulsatilla*, the mental state is different. The child feels weepy, helpless, whiny and demanding. There can often be yellow/green discharge from the ear or nose. The pain is often worse in a warm room and is better in the open air.

Sulphur should be considered when other remedies have not totally worked or you simply don't feel yourself. There is a lack of energy and interest. There may be some burning and pressure in the ear.

COMBINATION STRATEGY   If the symptoms are intense, acute, and there is a general fever, you can combine *Aconite*, *Chamomilla* and *Belladonna*, one tablet of each in two to four ounces of water, one tsp. taken every fifteen to sixty minutes until relief sets in. Follow with *Sulphur* if this does not work. *Hepar sulph* and *Mercurius* can also be mixed if you cannot make a distinction.

Use garlic/mullein ear oil, putting into the ear following instructions on the bottle. Plantago tincture may also be used.

Ear Injury

One should be very careful when dealing with any injury in the ear. Do not poke or put anything into the ear. One can easily injure the ear drum, even leading to perforation. If a drum is perforated, then also putting anything into the ear can lead to infection. If a foreign object is in the ear get professional attention. If this is not available, apply a gentle syringing of warm water with *Calendula* tincture added. Do not syringe directly into the center of the ear, but toward the top and let the liquid go down into the ear. If there is an abrasion to parts of the canal leading to the eardrum, wash carefully with warm water and *Calendula* and use *Calendula* cream after. Be very careful if putting *Calendula* on with a Q tip. If there is excessive wax in the ear, you can use a little mullein oil warmed on a hot spoon and gently put into the ear over a number of days to loosen the wax. For any pain in the ear, or anxiety consider giving *Aconite* or *Chamomilla*.

Eye Conditions

Blepharitis

Blepharitis in an infection of the margins of the eyelids. Although it can be an acute condition, it often recurs in a more chronic condition and requires constitutional homeopathic care to treat effectively.

Conjunctivitis

Conjunctivitis is a bacterial infection in the conjunctiva (the lining) of the eye. It may be the consequence of allergies and other irritations to the eye. Children often get this condition, called 'pinkeye'. It is mostly treated with topical antibiotics. It tends to be highly infectious.
See Chapter Fourteen: Trachoma

Styes and Chalazae

A stye is an inflamed lump/tumor found near the edge of the eyelid caused by a bacterial infection, often in the root of an eyelash. It can arise as an acute condition but often has a recurring chronic tendency. Symptoms are mainly an inflammation of the upper and/or lower eyelid, with swelling redness and itching. There are often hard nodules on the eyelid. A chalazion is a lump on the eyelid due to a blocked oil gland. It is normally larger than a stye, it doesn't hurt but can impede vision if large. It will normally go away of itself in time. A stye tends to be more toward the edge of the eyelid.

● **GENERAL CARE**

With conjunctivitis wash the eye well with warm water. Avoid contagion by washing hands frequently. Use homeopathic or other natural eye drops with *Euphrasia* (eyebright) in to help with the infection. With styes and chalazion, use warm compresses a few times a day. This may help open the pores, relieving the symptoms. Don't squeeze the stye or chalazion to try and open it. For babies with conjunctivitis, use breast milk.

◆ **HOMEOPATHIC CARE**

The first remedy for simple conjunctivitis is *Euphrasia*. Symptoms are burning and swelling of eyes and eyelids. There may be yellow and/or watery discharge from the eyes. *Pulsatilla* is also indicated for thick yellow/green discharge from the eyes. This is useful for children who are weepy, mild and clingy when sick. It is also a good remedy for simple styes, especially if found near the inner corner of the eyes. If there is a blocked tear duct, which is not uncommon in new born babies, leading to yellowy/green discharge from the eye, you can try *Pulsatilla* or *Silicea* if that doesn't work. If it persists, you should seek professional care.

Allium cepa can be given when there is excessive watering of the eyes and burning pain, but the discharge is bland. There can be great sensitivity to the light. *Belladonna* can be used when the eyes are very red, congested, with burning, fullness and great heat. The pupils are dilated. *Staphysagria* is given more for blepharitis occurring with styes or chalazae. The styes are hard and there are nodules on the lids which are itching. If a stye comes after an emotional upset or quarrel, then this is a good remedy. *Sulphur* is given when there is burning and dryness in the eye and it feels inflamed and swollen and may itch a lot, especially in a warm room.

✎ HERBAL CARE

Using an eye tincture of *Euphrasia* (eyebright) and/or *Hamamelis* (witch-hazel) is very good.

Eye Injury

● HOMEOPATHIC CARE

Arnica is the first remedy to give for a simple black eye, due to injury. If that doesn't clear everything up and bruising and swelling remain, you should give *Ledum*. *Ledum* is also useful for any injury due to a pointed object in the eye. *Symphytum* is useful for injury to the bone around the eye. It also follows *Arnica* well. Any serious injury to the eye and the face, including the bones of the face and skull should be checked as soon as possible by a medical expert. There may be a skull fracture.

If there is any foreign body in the eye, the eye can be bathed in an eyebath using three drops of either *Calendula*, *Hamamelis* or *Hypericum* tincture. For any pain or inflammation in the eye, from an object, injury or otherwise, *Euphrasia* (or similar eye mixture that has *Euphrasia* as one of the ingredients) should be used as an eyebath. *Euphrasia* in a 6c or 30c homeopathic potency can be used at the same time.

For simple eyestrain due to overexertion of using the eyes, perhaps reading in the dark or doing really fine work, then use *Ruta grav*, three times a day for three days.

Mouth Ulcers

These are common conditions which at times are more constitutional in nature and require more chronic treatment. However, they can come due to dietary factors as well as acute stress. Abscesses are different from

ulcers as they discharge pus and are found mainly on the gums.
See Toothache section and Chapter Twelve: Skin Conditions, Boils

● HOMEOPATHIC CARE

Borax is one of main remedies for small ulcers, commonly called aphthae, which children can often get. Children are often weepy and clingy and dislike being put down. They can have a fear of falling and therefore cling onto their parents. They have a fear of sudden noises. The aphthae can bleed easily and the mouth may have offensive taste and breath. *Mercurius* is the other main remedy to consider for mouth ulcers, often associated with an increase in salivation, especially at night, and a peculiar metallic or offensive taste in the mouth. If the ulcers are particular painful, with sharp pains and much salivation and offensive breath and perhaps cracks in the tongue or corner of the mouth, then *Nitric acid* is very good.

● HERBAL CARE

Golden seal tincture gargled in the mouth is effective. Repeat three times daily. Also clove oil can be used and is very soothing.

Sinusitis

Sinusitis is an infection of the sinus cavities, mostly felt in the nose, cheeks and forehead, although it can be felt in the back of the head also. Often it occurs due to an initial cold which leads to a secondary infection. Sometimes it is a chronic condition which mostly requires more constitutional treatment. However, in acute situations it can be effectively treated.

● GENERAL CARE

Using a netty pot to clear the sinuses with saline water is an effective way to prevent sinusitis and also to help clear the sinuses of infected mucus. Sometimes this is enough to cure a simple sinusitis. These can be bought at certain pharmacies and health food stores.

◆ **HOMEOPATHIC CARE**

Kali bichromicum is the most specific remedy for sinusitis when there are symptoms of great pressure in the sinuses, especially felt at the root of the nose and in the cheeks. Often you feel obstructed in the nose but nothing comes out when blowing it, or there is thick, stringy mucus that is hard to detach. There can also be profuse sticky mucus going down the back of the throat. *Belladonna* is good when acute sinusitis is attached to a fever and there is heat and throbbing in the sinuses and face, with much congestion.

🌿 **HERBAL CARE**

Golden seal should be taken by holding it in the mouth. Essential oils such as pine, tea tree and/or thyme can be taken as inhalations when mixed with hot water and the steam inhaled.

Teething

Teething is a normal development in a child but often during teething a child can become very upset emotionally and also it can have more general effects for the child. At times a child can get diarrhea when teething. Remedies such as *Chamomilla*, *Belladonna*, *Borax*, *Ipecac*, *Magnesium phosphoricum* and *Silicea* can be thought of. At times it requires more constitutional treatment and can be part of other develop-ment issues in a child, such as late developing walking or talking and in those cases *Calcarea carbonica* and *Silicea* are two of the main remedies. Often the child needing *Calcarea carbonica* is more chubby and sweaty, while *Silicea* is more thin, fragile looking but also sweaty.

◆ **HOMEOPATHIC CARE**

The first remedy to consider for teething, when the child is easily upset, weepy, irritable and very contrary is *Chamomilla*. Often children want to be picked up and carried and then put down again. Nothing can satisfy them. A child can ask for food and then throw it away. It can drive the parent to distraction. *Borax* is needed if the child wants to be carried all the time and has a fear of being put down. If *Chamomilla* doesn't work, give *Borax*. The child may also have apthae (sores) in the mouth. *Ipecac* is needed if there is vomiting associated with teething and *Magnesium phosphoricum* if there is abdominal cramping.

Throat Conditions

This includes all forms of sore throat, tonsillitis, laryngitis, lost voice etc. Many of the remedies recommended can be found for many other types of infections. A sore throat often comes with other more general symptoms, a fever, a general cold, influenza or bronchitis. However, some people simply get a sore throat once a year, which is relatively mild. Only treat it if it is limiting, painful or it can lead to something worse. One of the most dangerous throat infections is diphtheria but is rarely seen nowadays. If traveling in developing countries, it is possible it would be seen and should be suspected if the sore throat is extremely intense, with fever and chill, difficulty breathing, foul bloody nasal discharge and enlarged lymph glands in the neck. It can be treated with antibiotics. Children can often get sore throats with inflammation of tonsils.

See Chapter Seven: Common Infections, Chapter Eight: Colds and Coughs, Chapter Fourteen: Other Tropical and Infectious Diseases, Diphtheria

● **GENERAL CARE**

As with any infection, including colds, keeping warm is important and this is especially the case with throat conditions. Wrap the neck up and drink warm drinks. Sucking lozenges may give relief but don't do it the same time as taking a remedy. Don't strain the voice if the larynx and trachea are affected.

● **HOMEOPATHIC CARE**

Belladonna is one of the best remedies for simple tonsillitis and throat inflammation when it is sudden, intense and associated with burning and fever. There is an affinity for the right side of the throat. The tongue can look red and shiny. *Hepar sulph* and *Mercurius* are two of the best remedies for inflamed throat and tonsillitis when there are sharp, stitching pains in the throat, extending into the ears when swallowing.

Hepar sulph especially is useful when it feels like a needle or splinter is in the throat and the pain is often better from warm liquids and wrapping up the throat. It is much worse from cold liquids. There may be a hoarse voice. *Mercurius* is needed when there is often an offensive taste in the mouth, mostly metallic, insipid or just bad, with a yellow coating of the tongue. Often there is an increased salivation, even dribbling on the pillow at night. There can be trembling of the tongue when it is protruded.

Phytolacca is a good remedy for simple sore throats, especially when the lymph glands of the neck are swollen and tender, for which *Mercurius* is also indicated. Tonsils are swollen and red, and the neck is stiff. Symptoms are often better when cold drinks are taken and become worse from warmth.

Lachesis is useful when the left side of the throat is mostly affected, and there is a feeling of a lump in the throat. There is difficulty in swallowing, especially liquids, whereas solids are easier. *Arum tryphillum* is used when there is great rawness of the throat with a lost voice, the pain worse from coughing or clearing the throat. *Rhus tox* is good for a simple lost voice from using the voice too much or exposure to cold weather. *Argentum nitricum* is useful when you lose your voice before having to perform or give a talk, a form of anticipatory anxiety.

NOTE It is not always easy to find the correct remedy. Try one and if it does not work in one to two days, try another. If it is a simple sore throat with no discernible symptoms, try *Phytolacca* first and follow with *Mercurius* if needed.

Toothache

A toothache always needs to be checked with a dentist to find out the reason for the pain. However, using homeopathic remedies can relieve the pain and at times deal with the whole situation. Be careful when having dental work in places where the quality cannot be guaranteed. When you have an abscess of the gums, it may be due to a simple infection, which can happen when traveling and when coming across more unusual bacteria. It can also indicate a deeper problem in the roots of the teeth. If that is so, dentists mostly will recommend a root canal.

However, if traveling, it is best to treat the infection, either with antibiotics and or homeopathic remedies and after that get the tooth looked at when you get home. Some dentists can want to do root canals very quickly when perhaps the body will take care of the problem itself. If you really do need a root canal, the body will tell you as the abscess or pain will come back. It is often not an emergency and the situation should be reviewed once the infection is cleared up. This is both when traveling and when at home. Find a dentist you can really trust.

See Chapter Four: Accidents, Injuries and Trauma, Pain section

● GENERAL CARE

Taking pain killers as necessary and also using cloves to help to numb the area can help. Do not take at the same time as a homeopathic remedy as it may antidote the remedy. If there is an abscess in the gums, keep the mouth very clean. Gargle with salt water and also use essential oils. See herbal care.

● HOMEOPATHIC CARE

A homeopathic remedy can work quickly to relieve the pain if the underlying problem is not severe. The pain will be relieved in minutes to a couple of hours, depending on the severity of the pain. *Chamomilla* is the first remedy for teething children who are irritable and capricious and who have colic and/or diarrhea from teething. It can also be used for general tooth pain but *Coffea* is the first remedy to consider for severe pain. There is great sensitivity in the teeth, which is worse from all stimulation, noises etc. The pain is worse from touch and chewing and better from ice water in the mouth. You are not able to sleep because of the pain. Use *Nux vomica* when there is great pain with sensitivity to all stimuli and a feeling of great irritability with the pain. Also consider Magnesium phos for teething and teeth pains which are better from warmth and pressure.

For abscess of the gums, the main remedies are *Hepar sulph*, *Mercurius* and *Silicea*, similar to when given for abscesses of the skin. *Hepar sulph* is needed for very painful abscesses with sharp, stitching pains; *Mercurius* when there is a painful abscess, with increased saliva and at times a foul, or metallic taste in the mouth. There may be swelling of the cheek on the affected side. *Silicea* is more often needed if the problem is a recurrent one and if there is any discharge from the abscess. *Staphysagria* is also useful for abscesses when it recurs and also when there is decaying of the roots or crown of the teeth, and blackening of the teeth. *Hekla lava* is indicated when there is hard swelling of the jaw with a large abscess.

See Chapter Twelve: Skin Conditions, Boils

COMBINATION STRATEGY If you are not sure which remedy is needed, mix one tablet of *Hepar sulph* and *Mercurius* into two to four ounces of water and take one tsp. three to five times daily.

HERBAL CARE

Taking cloves may be useful in helping toothache. Other essential oils, such as eucalyptus, peppermint, oregano and wintergreen oils can be used, rubbing into the gums and/or putting onto a toothbrush and brushing into teeth and gums. This is especially when there is an abscess as it helps to maintain good oral hygiene.

Chapter Ten
Women's Conditions

Breast and Vaginal Issues

This may include inflammation of the breast (mastitis) due to breast feeding problems, or other breast feeding issues. For breast abscesses, also refer to Chapter Twelve: Skin Conditions, Boils section. For injuries to the breast, also look at Chapter Four: Accidents, Injuries and Trauma. If lumps remain after a significant blow to the breast or there is bleeding from the nipple for any reason, seek medical advice.

For acute vaginal herpetic eruptions or candida, a topical use of neem oil mixed with yoghurt and olive oil can help. Internal homeopathic remedies such as *Rhus tox* or *Dulcamara* can be given for an acute herpetic eruption, but constitutional care is ideally needed.
Also see Chapter Seven: Common Infections

● HOMEOPATHIC CARE

For acute inflammation of the breast, when there is great heat, redness and burning, and the pain is worse from any motion, then *Belladonna* is the remedy. If there is hardness in the breast, along with heat, but not as intense as *Belladonna* and where any motion makes it worse, *Bryonia* is needed. If the breast is extremely hard, perhaps with nodules and pain and swelling extends into the armpit and the nipples may be cracked, *Phytolacca* is needed.

In simple blocked ducts when breast feeding, *Phytolacca* is the first remedy to give where there is any hardness of the breast. It is also the first remedy for abscesses in the breasts that are complications of mastitis and/or blocked ducts. There can be painful cracks in the nipples. *Urtica urens* is needed when milk decreases or stops in one breast, with no other symptoms. *Pulsatilla* is needed if there is much weepiness and emotion along with problems with breast feeding. There may be not enough milk or after weaning the child, the milk continues. There may be an increased desire to walk in the open air, or simply for fresh air. *Silicea* may be needed (for the mother) if the baby refuses to take the milk or vomits after feeding. It seems the milk is not good for the child. There can be sharp pains in the breasts and inflammation and hardness of the breast.

For any injury to the breast, especially when involving a blow which leaves a lump, *Bellis perennis* can be used. It is similar to *Arnica* and from the same botanical family. Use *Arnica* if you don't have *Bellis perennis*. Another remedy for residual lumps in the breast from blows is *Conium* but it is best to get professional homeopathic advice. For thrush on the nipples of nursing women when the baby also has thrush, take *Borax*.

🍃 HERBAL CARE

Vervaine (*Verbena officianalis*) can be given in tea form to help stimulate milk production, especially when feeling exhausted from too much stress and care. Nettle tea (*Urtica urens*) can also be given in tea form to do the same thing. Nettle is an amazing herb and is full of vitamins and minerals. Asafœtida tea promotes production of breast milk.

Menstrual Issues

Most menstrual problems require more constitutional care as they are mostly chronic in nature. However, in more acute situations or when away, the more immediate symptoms can be treated to give relief. For bleeding problems, also look at Chapter Four: Accidents, Injuries and

Trauma, Hemorrhage and Pain sections and the remedies for hemorrhage in the After Birth section below.

◆ HOMEOPATHIC CARE

For excessive cramping pains, you can consider *Chamomilla* when pains feel unbearable and when you feel angry. *Colocynthis* is needed when the pains double you up, and you want to press strongly into the abdomen. *Magnesium phosphoricum* has similar pains, with strong cramping and where pressure and also hot applications and rubbing give relief. The period may have come early with the pains. *Nux vomica* is given when there is great sensitivity to all impressions, great irritability and impatience. *Sepia* is needed when there is great bearing down pains, as if the uterus is going to come out and you have to sit down. You feel exhausted and irritable. For other remedies, look at the remedies indicated in labor situations.

Pregnancy and Birth

● GENERAL CARE

Pregnancy and birth are ideally joyful events but there are times when support is needed and remedies can help. If you are pregnant and going into labor, then please get someone to help you if you need to find a remedy. Give them the book to use. If there is a risk of a miscarriage or you feel you are going into labor and are not in the right place and are not ready, then you can find a remedy while you are getting prepared.

If you are a helper looking for a remedy to give, please read the following information:

Remedies in pregnancy and especially in labor may be given or repeated frequently, one tablet every five to fifteen minutes until you see change. If there is no change in one hour in intense situations, you should look to change the remedy. Let her find a comfortable position – lying on one's back is often the worst. *Nux vomica* is a useful remedy to take if you (the helper) faint at the sight of blood. Also, if you are feeling stressed and anxious take Rescue Remedy, the Bach Flower remedy. Give it to the mother-to-be as well if she is anxious. Also, advise her to open her mouth in a big round O. It is like opening the cervix; it helps.

After the birth lay the baby skin-to-skin on the mother's chest and then cover them with a warmed soft piece of clothing or sheet. Wait for the placenta. It should come within twenty minutes. Watch out for hemorrhage. When the placenta is delivered, check that it is intact and not broken. The caul (birth membrane) should be shiny like petrol on water. Give *Ipecac* if you think there is a lot of blood. (It always looks a lot if you are not used to midwifery). Make sure there are scissors in the first aid kit, to cut the clamped cord (use clothes pegs, elastic band, hair tie, dental floss but don't pull too tight or it will slice the cord). Sterilize the scissors first by pouring boiling water over them. Otherwise clamp the cord and bite it free after it has finished pulsating. Women give birth so few times in their lives, so it should ideally be an occasion of celebration and joy.

Nausea

◆ HOMEOPATHIC CARE

Nausea normally happens during the first trimester (three months) of pregnancy. Often it is mild but at times can be very debilitating and for some women it extends into the second trimester of pregnancy. One of the first remedies to consider is *Sepia*. It is indicated when there is nausea and vomiting, which is often worse from the smell and/or sight of food. Often one feels emotionally flat, even irritable, with no energy at all. It is a useful remedy when the woman feels ambivalent about being pregnant. *Nux vomica* is another good remedy when nausea is combined with intense retching or there is real difficulty to vomit, even if the urge is there. There is often an extreme sensitivity to smells, including food, and irritability is again a factor. *Tabacum* is needed when there is intense nausea with a great sinking feeling in the stomach, vertigo and a feeling as if the nausea is 'deathly'. It feels unbearable, with great weakness. *Lactic acid* is another good remedy in serious and extended nausea when there is much salivation with the nausea and weakness. If there is much salivation and *Lactic acid* doesn't work, then *Kreosotum* can be tried. *Ipecac* is another strong nausea remedy, with intense vomiting which feels uncontrollable and again there can be much salivation. There is great exhaustion and the stomach feels as if it is empty and and hanging.

Miscarriage

The threat of miscarriage is something that can happen to anyone during pregnancy. For some women it is a much greater risk than for others, and all precautions need to be taken. Traveling during these times should be avoided if you are at risk of miscarrying. A miscarriage can happen at any time during the pregnancy but is more likely to occur in the first three to five months. There are many possible remedies in this situation and the following are just a few options. Professional homeopathic and medical advice should be sought if it seems a miscarriage is possible. It is important to see if there are any causes that may risk a miscarriage, including shock, grief, physical trauma etc. If that is clear, look at remedies that cover these causes. Many of the same remedies indicated for possible miscarriage will be indicated during normal labor so it is useful to read the whole section.

● HOMEOPATHIC CARE

If the threat of miscarriage starts after too much physical exertion, immediately take *Arnica*, in a 30c or 200c, putting one tablet in a glass of water and taking one sip every fifteen minutes for up to four hours. If it is due to strong emotional shock, take *Aconite* in the same way. If that doesn't work follow up with *Gelsemium*. *Sepia* is one of the first remedies to consider, especially when there is a strong dragging down feeling in the uterine region which feels much better when sitting down and crossing the legs. *Caulophyllum* is an important remedy in homeopathy for labor and birth issues, including miscarriages. It has symptoms of intense, erratic contractions that seem to fly about the body. The person can feel very overexcited and irritable. *Ipecac* is indicated if contractions come from excessive nausea and vomiting.

Vibernum is a great remedy when there are strong contractions that extend down the front of the thighs and that can come from the back. Other remedies to consider are *Belladonna*, *Chamomilla*, *Gelsemium* and *Sabina*. *Sabina* is indicated often when there is a tendency to miscarry in the first trimester and when pains move from the sacrum (lower back) to the front of the pubic region and back again and also pains shoot up the vagina. There can be great nervousness and sensitivity, especially to music. See below for other remedy descriptions.

Labor and Birth

Ideally this should be a natural process, without complication, but for many reasons this isn't always the case and homeopathic remedies can help. It is well known that complications arise when in stressed situations, which modern hospital environments can induce, and where recourse to caesarian sections are done much too quickly. Difficulties in labor therefore can have both physical and psychological causes and when choosing a remedy, attention needs to be given to both areas. There are also midwives who specialize in using homeopathy during pregnancy and labor and it is important to have all the support you can during this important time.

◆ HOMEOPATHIC CARE

One of the complications of labor is called a 'rigid os', which is when the cervix does not dilate, for whatever reason. This tends to stop or inhibit the natural contractions leading up to birth. For all problems in the labor process the main remedies to consider are *Caulophyllum*, *Chamomilla*, *Cimicifuga*, *Gelsemium*, *Kali carbonicum*, *Pulsatilla* and *Sepia*. If there is great fright and shock, then also consider *Aconite* if there is fear that she or the baby will die and *Ignatia* if she feels emotionally out of control and weepy. Look at how the woman is dealing with it. If she feels exhausted and wants to give up, think of *Caulophyllum* and *Sepia*. If angry and screaming, think of *Chamomilla* and *Cimicifuga*. *Gelsemium* in particular is strong when she is feeling very frightened and anxious that she can't go through with it. *Natrum muriaticum* is good when the woman feels too many people are around and wants to be alone. *Pulsatilla* is excellent when the cervix is dilated at 7cm but won't go any further and if there are no other symptoms to indicate another remedy. *Sepia* is useful when there are intense bearing down pains, felt in both the uterus and back region. One important condition in late pregnancy is a breech birth when the baby is not in the right position. If this is the case, *Pulsatilla* is the first remedy to give. Give one tablet every fifteen minutes to every hour if in the midst of labor or every four hours for one to two days if before in full labor. A change should be seen in one to four hours if the situation is acute or up to one day if less urgent.

In the midst of labor, if contractions tend to become erratic and weak, consider *Caulophyllum*. This is often the first remedy to consider. *Cimicifuga* is also important, especially when there is great sensitivity to noise and pains are moving about a lot, going from ovary to ovary or moving down the thighs and emotionally feeling weepy, depressed and frustrated. *Pulsatilla* also has similar symptoms but often there is much weeping and a feeling of great helplessness. She wants people around and craves open air, wanting all windows open. In *Chamomilla* there is anger and pains are unendurable. *Coffea* is similar to *Chamomilla*. Don't forget *Arnica* if the woman feels bruised and sore all over and she can't get comfortable as the bed feels too hard. In *Kali carbonicum*, the labor is felt mainly in the back, as if it is weak and about to break, with weak labor pains which extend down the legs, similar to *Cimicifuga* and *Viburnum*.

When contractions seem to suddenly cease totally, the main remedies to consider are again *Belladonna*, *Chamomilla*, *Caulophyllum*, *Cimicifuga*, *Kali carbonicum*, *Pulsatilla* and *Sepia*. See their descriptions above. If you can't decide which remedy to give, mix one tablet of each remedy you are considering into a glass of water and sip once every five to fifteen minutes until you notice some change. Stir the mixture each time you take a sip. Also remedies for bleeding may be needed, which are discussed below.

After Birth

● HOMEOPATHIC CARE

A couple of important issues after birth are retained placenta and unnatural bleeding that doesn't stop. For the first condition, you can consider *Arnica*, *Belladonna*, *Cantharis*, *Caulophyllum Cimicifuga*, *Gelsemium*, *Nux vomica*, *Pulsatilla*, *Sabina* and *Sepia*. As with many homeopathic conditions, there is one particular remedy that will work best but others may also work to some extent. If you are not clear which remedy to give, try *Arnica* first and then *Pulsatilla*. The placenta can take up to 20 minutes to appear after birth. If there is great exhaustion and weakness give *Gelsemium*. If much irritability and spasmodic pains, give *Nux vomica*; if much weepiness, give *Pulsatilla*. If there are strong urinary symptoms at the same time and much burning, give *Cantharis*. If there is also much bleeding and shooting pains up the vagina, give *Sabina*. Don't forget to consider *Aconite* if there is any shock after birth, with fear, anxiety and shivering.

For general increased bleeding after birth, give *Arnica* to begin with, because of the trauma involved. If that doesn't work, consider *Ipecac* if there is much bright blood and especially if there is nausea with the bleeding. Consider *Sabina* if there are many clots with the bleeding, *China* if there is great weakness from loss of blood, *Hamamelis* if there is constant, dark flow after a long traumatic birth, and also other remedies described before, such as *Belladonna* if the blood feels hot and is intense and pulsating and *Gelsemium* if there is great weakness. Two other smaller remedies to consider are *Thlaspi bursa pastoris* and *Ustilago*. With the first remedy there may or may not be violent colicky pains with the bleeding. With *Ustilago*, the bleeding is quite passive with clots and it may be ropy in quality.

See Chapter four, Accidents, Injuries and Trauma, Hemorrhage section

Some women suffer from post natal depression after birth. This can come on even months later. In most cases, this requires constitutional homeopathic treatment. However, if there is some depression and a feeling of being under a dark cloud or feeling that you are caged in by the new responsibilities of motherhood, take *Cimicifuga*, twice daily for five days. If you feel weepy and need a lot of consolation all the time, take *Pulsatilla*. If symptoms continue, seek professional care.

🌿 HERBAL CARE

Shepherds Purse (*Thlaspi bursa pastoris*) Tincture to 6x. This is good for uterine hemorrhage, with cramps and colic, whether from a miscarriage, labor and post labor. Follow instructions on the label.

Chapter Eleven
Bladder And Kidneys

Cystitis

Cystitis is an infection of the bladder, due to a bacterial infection. It may be caused by having sex, by being unable to wash frequently, by heat, or it can be due to a more chronic vulnerability. In the latter case, constitutional homeopathic care is needed. It is important to see if there is any pain in the mid back region, which could indicate the infection going to the kidney. See Kidney section. If that is the case, seek medical attention. At times, the infection can begin in the kidney. In an acute kidney infection, one should see relief from fever and pain in about two to three hours. If there is no change in four hours, in any way, choose another remedy. If there is some change, even if slight, continue with the remedy. In cystitis, improvement may take longer but some change should be seen between four hours and one day, depending on the severity of the symptoms.

● GENERAL CARE

At the first sign of symptoms, drink a lot of water. Cranberry juice is often used as well and seems to help avert the condition. Avoid alcohol and acidic drinks. Symptoms are usually a combination of an increased urging to urinate, burning pain in the urethra before, during and/or after urination, occasional fever, general sick feeling, aching in the bladder and back pain. The urine may be cloudy, bloody, with an offensive odor. The urging to urinate may be very intense, but with little urine being passed.

If you develop blood in the urine or begin to suffer from cystitis, kidney stones, prostate or uterine infections and have spent time in Africa and other tropical regions within two years, then Bilharzia should be considered.

See Chapter Fourteen: Other Tropical and Infectious Diseases, Bilharzia

● HOMEOPATHIC CARE

For simple cystitis that comes from having sex, you should first take *Staphysagria*. If you develop very intense symptoms, very quickly, with a violent, constant urging, but only a few drops are passed, or the urine is bloody, then you should take *Cantharis*. It is also needed if the infection goes into the kidneys. *Berberis* is needed when you have pains in the kidneys along with the cystitis with pains radiating outwards from the bladder region and often extending down the legs and to the kidneys. Pains are always changing place. *Berberis* is needed when the kidney is the primary area affected with burning pains and pains radiating down toward the bladder and into the back. It is one of the first remedies for kidney stones with intense colicky pains. *Lycopodium* is a good kidney colic remedy, when the right side is affected and there is red sand in the urine. There may be abdominal symptoms seen, which is described in Chapter Six: Digestive Conditions, Hepatitis section. *Equisetum* is a good cystitis remedy when the strongest symptom is simply a great fullness in the bladder which is not relieved when urinating. *Nux vomica* is needed if you have an intense, cutting, violent, stitching pain in the kidney region, and you have a strong urging to urinate but little passes. It is also a kidney colic remedy. It sounds similar to *Cantharis*, but the symptoms indicating *Cantharis* are even more intense and frenzied and there is more blood in the urine.

If none of the other remedies seem indicated or haven't worked, then you should try *Sarsaparilla*. It is one of the most indicated remedies in cystitis. Often, the burning pain is felt right at the end of urination and there can be a chill feeling spreading up the urethra to the bladder. You may have the strange experience of feeling gas pass from the bladder. *Apis* is an important remedy for acute kidney infection (nephritis), especially when it comes on suddenly, with great burning, stinging and a fever but with no thirst. You may see a strange puffiness around the eyelids. There can a bursting feeling in the bladder and kidney, with fullness of the bladder and hot urine. *Belladonna* is needed when cystitis comes on very quickly and intensely, with burning and a hot, dry fever. Pains are often throbbing and the urine is also burning.

See Chapter Seven: Common Infections

COMBINATION STRATEGY If in doubt as to which remedy to give, put one tablet of each remedy that seems indicated into a glass of water, and sip the glass frequently (every fifteen to thirty minutes depending on the severity of symptoms). Stir the water before taking each sip. For a kidney infection, if no remedy is clear, use *Apis*, *Berberis*, *Cantharis* and *Nux vomica* together. Put one tablet of each remedy in a glass of water and take a sip every ten minutes until some relief is felt, stirring the water each time. Change should be noticed in one to two hours.

✦ HERBAL CARE

Take one or more of the following, either in a tea or tincture: Uva ursi, dandelion leaf, marshmallow root, juniper root or horsetail. Goldenrod is also very useful. Cranberry can be taken, either in juice form or tablets. It is useful to prevent a urinary infection get any worse.

Kidney Disease

Inflammation of the kidneys is a potentially serious condition and requires immediate medical treatment if possible. It can stem from a bladder infection which then moves to the kidney or may be due to a blockage in one of the ureters (the tubes coming from the kidney and going to the bladder). Stones coming from the kidney can get stuck in the ureter leading to excruciating pain. Kidney infections may be due to some underlying vulnerability in the region. Kidney stones tend to begin with sudden, intense pain, and without fever or burning urination. A kidney stone may require surgical intervention and needs to be medically diagnosed.

● GENERAL CARE

Especially in kidney stones, one should drink a lot of fluid. Ideally this will help pass the kidney stone.

● HOMEOPATHIC CARE

See Cystitis Section

● HERBAL CARE

Take goldenrod in tincture form three drops three times a day.

Chapter Twelve
Skin Conditions

There are many skin conditions, some of which accompany other illnesses mentioned in the book and need to be studied with those conditions. When traveling and at home, there are some conditions seen which are due to a combination of being in intense heat or from poor hygiene, dirty hotels etc. These are either fungal or parasite infections. Hygiene is the key to prevention, but at times they can't be avoided.

When traveling, the skin can take a hammering, from too much sun, with difficulties in hygiene, the feet drying out from wearing flip flops leading to cracking and pain, and various skin infections that easily come from scratches and slight wounds. Take a good soap with you, ideally a liquid soap that is easily portable. Soaps in more basic areas are often not nice and can cause local allergic reactions.

● GENERAL CARE

Maintaining good skin is important. Using a ripe avocado is one natural way to nourish the skin, mashing up the avocado and applying immediately. It can be left for hours or overnight. Using good oil on the skin may help. Coconut oil and other vegetable oils can be used. Clean your feet regularly and rub rough skin off around the heel to prevent drying and cracking and apply oil. For irritating skin conditions of all sorts, putting raw cabbage on the affected area can relieve. This is useful especially for children who are itching intensely at irritated parts. Loosely bandage the cabbage to the irritated part and change daily.

Animals: Lice, Fleas and Bedbugs

Lice fleas and bedbugs are one of the unfortunate consequences of travel and of sleeping in infected beds all over the world. Lice most commonly occur due to poor hygiene and can be more easily avoided. The most commonly seen are head lice, often afflicting children and easily spread. Lice can also be found in the groin and pubic region and are known as crabs. Body lice can be carriers of diseases such as typhus and relapsing fever. Typhus used to be an epidemic disease in times of war and extreme hardship, e.g., prisons and concentration camps. Millions in human history have died as a result of the bacterial infection from lice but in modern times and when traveling, it is generally not seen. There is a vaccine and antibiotic therapy is effective. For relapsing fever see Chapter Fifteen, Tick bite diseases.

Body lice can be spread easily from one person to another and pubic lice through sex. Head lice do not carry these diseases. Head lice are recognized by their nits, pale little balls often seen in the margins of the hair, especially the neck. They are difficult to remove. These nits should be removed, either with a nit comb or even by shaving the head if necessary.

● GENERAL CARE

Using coconut oil on the head after washing can help remove the nits. Tea tree oil can also be used to help kill the nits. One problem commonly found is that although the lice can be removed, enough nits remain to re-infect the person, so all nits have to be removed. Treatment needs to be done for at least one week to prevent re-infection. Body lice can be treated in a similar way, using tea tree oil mixed with bathing water and washed onto the skin. Fleas and bed bugs are also common, bed bugs being commonly found in unclean hotels and even in higher class places all over the world. With bed bugs, washing all infected clothing and linens is essential.

◗ HOMEOPATHIC CARE

Bites may be painful but are often just very itchy. If bites become very irritating, *Staphysagria* may be tried, three times a day for up to three days. It can also be used for head lice.

◢ HERBAL CARE

Tea tree oil can be used to help with bites and also to prevent being bitten. Other sprays such as pyrethrum can be used.

Boils and Abscesses

Boils are often caused by a bacterial infection, often affecting a hair follicle or due to broken skin becoming infected. If left untreated, they can either erupt or become re-absorbed into the body. A carbuncle is a large boil which is abscessing, often with more than one opening, draining pus onto the skin. The same remedies are needed as with a boil, but it needs to be kept very clean to prevent further infection. A bad carbuncle may need professional medical attention to see what underlying condition may be the primary cause. Recurrent boils or abscesses can also require constitutional treatment once the acute symptoms are controlled.

Abscesses may develop from a boil or be an expression on the skin of a deeper infection in the body, the abscess being a vent for the infection. Once an abscess has burst, it is important to keep it clean and to give appropriate remedies for the abscess and the underlying infection. Abscesses also occur on the gums of the mouth, often due to an underlying infection of the roots of the teeth. The same remedies described below can be used.

● GENERAL CARE

Do not burst a boil. Let it take its own course. Once it has burst, keep clean, wash in warm water and use *Calendula* tincture (diluted in some water). Alternatively use *Echinacea* tincture. Ensure the water is boiled first.

● HOMEOPATHIC CARE

There are two main remedies when the boil or abscess is threatening to burst and needs either to be reabsorbed or brought to the surface. *Hepar sulph* is needed when the boils/abscesses have a sharp, stitching pain and are much worse for touch and cold air. It can feel as though there is a splinter there. *Silicea* is the other remedy for abscesses or boils that don't heal quickly. Both are good remedies for abscesses of the gums. *Silicea* can follow *Hepar sulph* if that remedy doesn't complete the situation and it is good to help finally heal a chronic abscess that isn't healing fully. *Hekla lava* is also a good remedy for abscesses in the gums when the other remedies don't work and when the abscess is hard and the jaw is swollen and painful. (This remedy was found when an English doctor noticed that cows feeding on grass around Mt Hekla in Iceland developed bony growths on their jaws).

If the boil is very inflamed and burning with redness and pressure and it comes on very quickly then *Belladonna* is the remedy needed. There is often great heat and/or stinging. Once it has become an abscess and there is burning and becoming a purple color and looks as if it is becoming infected, then *Lachesis* is needed. There may be throbbing and discharge of thin, bloody pus. If the boil threatens to turn into a carbuncle and become more deeply infected, with great burning, then *Tarentula cubensis* can be given. If an abscess has developed into a more general systemic infection with classic symptoms of blood poisoning – fever, chill, restlessness, achiness of the body, a rapid pulse but with low temperature, then *Pyrogen* can be given but medical attention should be sought.

● HERBAL CARE

Make a clay pack as for bites. Take *Echinacea* tincture, ten drops per hour for four to six hours. Repeat daily for three to five days. Make a hot compress using two drops of tea tree and lavender oil and apply to the area. Also apply neat lavender to the area.

Chilblains

Chilblains are due to a problem with the blood flow to the extremities and exposure to cold weather. A contraction of veins or just bad circulation made worse in the cold creates congestion of blood in the exposed part leading to swelling, itching, redness and burning. It is not a very serious condition and some people are more inclined to get them than others.

● GENERAL CARE

Avoid allowing extremities to become overexposed to the cold. If already afflicted, do not expose to intense heat, but gradually warm the part. The most likely parts affected are the toes, fingers, ears and nose.

● HOMEOPATHIC CARE

Agaricus is the most specific remedy to give, similar to that of frostbite. *Pulsatilla* is useful when the itching is much worse from the heat, which is often the case and is more often needed as a constitutional remedy for the condition.

● HERBAL CARE

Rub tea tree oil onto the inflamed parts.

Fungal Infections

There are various forms of fungus (commonly called tinea), from one that affects the crotch area (crotch itch or dhobie itch) and classic ringworm (which is a fungal eruption creating round patterns of raised, red skin). It can also occur on the scalp, creating bald patches, and is mainly seen in children. In another form of skin fungus - tinea versicolor - one sees blotches of skin discoloration which look lighter or at times darker than the rest of the skin. Another fungus is commonly known as athletes' foot. This latter condition is extremely common, highly infectious and difficult to get rid of. One needs to treat it for up to one month continually and even then it can tend to return.

Another common fungal condition is candida. It can be found all over the body and often begins with little red dots that gets more red, raised and angry and gradually spread from the original outbreak. It is mostly found in the warm areas of the body, the armpits, crotch and under the breasts. It is often the cause of diaper rash in babies. Candida is also found in the genital region of women and also in the nipples of breast feeding women. Thrush is a form of candida commonly found in the mouths of babies. Candida albicans is a form of candida often found in the digestive tract and also the respiratory tract and genitalia. They are normally found there but at times they greatly increase in number, leading to local and systemic symptoms. It has been speculated in recent years that when people have chronic candida infections in the body it lead to other more chronic problems and much has been written about candida diets and other therapies to purge the candida from the body. In a healthy body, fungi should not be able to prosper. However, the abuse of antibiotics for generations, including the amount in the food supply, along with other external factors may be one reason why there has been a huge increase in fungal conditions of all sorts in recent years. For example, in those who are immune deficient, such as people who are HIV positive it is often seen that systemic fungal infections are found along with other conditions.

● **GENERAL CARE**

Keep the skin well-washed and in cases where the groin is affected, allow as much air as possible. There are many different natural external topical treatments that can be used. Some may work better than others, depending on the person and also the severity of the infection. Eat very little or no sugar. Even cut down on fruits to lower the amount of sugar in the system. Fungi thrive on sugar. Conventional anti-fungal treatments can be used on the skin if necessary.

◆ **HOMEOPATHIC CARE**

For babies with thrush, the two main remedies are *Borax* and *Mercurius*. See Chapter Nine: ENT, Mouth ulcers. For general thrush, more constitutional care is needed but local herbal applications can be effective as well as changing habits, such as diet and hygiene measures. For ring-worm, especially on the scalp, where there are thick crusts, moist and dry, and round patches of hair loss, you can use *Dulcamara*, giving it three times daily for up to one week. Other more chronic based remedies are *Calcarea carbonica*, *Graphites* and *Sulphur*. The first is used in young children, who are generally overweight and sweaty, especially about the head, and where the whole head may be covered with crusts. In *Graphites*, there is oozing of honey like liquid which then dries up and in *Sulphur*, there is insufferable itching, especially when they get warm.

🌿 HERBAL CARE

Tea tree oil and lavender are used to treat many types of tinea. They can be mixed with a neutral oil, like olive or almond oil and put onto the affected parts after washing. For tinea versicolor, using apple cider vinegar can work. Tea tree oil or garlic oil can be used for athlete's foot. Neem oil can also be used for all types of fungal infections, including vaginal candida, where it can be mixed with yoghurt or olive oil.

Hives

Hives are a type of urticarial eruption, often with swelling, redness, bumps and itching of the skin. It can come from an allergic reaction, usually to food, e.g., shellfish or some external irritant, e.g., pollen, or it can come from being stressed. The body releases too much histamine, resulting in a skin eruption. Hives can come from overexposure to the sun or simply due to sensitivity to the sun. This sensitivity can be induced by taking medications and other products, including using sun block! If possible, stop taking any offending product but even then it can take a while for any allergic reaction to subside.
See Chapter Nine: ENT, Allergies section

💧 HOMEOPATHIC CARE

Apis is one of the first remedies for hives when there is stinging, burning and redness of the skin, associated mostly with a general allergic reaction to some external stimuli, e.g., shellfish. Often there is swelling with the redness and may be seen on the face, especially around the eyes. *Urtica urens* is the other major remedy for hives which are caused by shellfish and has similar symptoms, especially great stinging of the skin. *Rhus tox* is the other major remedy for hives and looks very similar to *Apis*. All three remedies can be combined if necessary.

Impetigo

One other common condition found especially in children is the highly infectious bacterial disease, impetigo. It is mostly found on the face and consists of itchy, crusty eruptions, at times oozing sticky moisture. As it is infectious and can spread to other children quickly, antibiotic therapy is mostly given. It is good to keep your child away from others if he/she is affected and treat either with both homeopathy and conventional medicine.

◆ HOMEOPATHIC CARE

Antimonium crudum is one of the most important remedies for impetigo. There are crusty thick eruptions, both dry and moist and are found anywhere on the body, but especially the face. Mentally, children are often cross, peevish and averse to being looked at. *Rhus tox* is another remedy to consider when there are eruptions rather like shingles. *Mezereum* can also be given for impetigo. *Croton tiglium* is one other remedy to think of when there are thick, rough, crusty eruptions which burst. The skin can feel thick and rough. *Dulcamara* is useful when the eruptions are thick, crusty and become moist and perhaps have come on after exposure to cold and damp.

See Shingles Section

COMBINATION STRATEGY If you do not know which remedy to choose, put one tablet of all the remedies (or which ones you have access to) into four ounces of water, and give one tsp. three times daily for five to seven days. Stop giving it if symptoms either get better or worse.

Poison Oak/Ivy

This is an allergic skin condition due to exposure to various forms of the plant species of poison ivy or poison oak (*Rhus toxicodendrum, Rhus radicans, Rhus diversiloba,* etc.). It is very common in North America and is found in most rural and wooded areas. Some people are highly allergic and will have a strong local and systemic reaction, affecting all parts of the body, including the genitalia and face, and even the throat. Other people seem virtually immune to it. Often it happens that a dog which has been walking in the woods will spread the resin from the plant to humans. If there is any suspicion of exposure, the skin must be washed very well, along with clothing, and products used to ensure that all the oil is off the body. Many people say different things work for them. Just a small amount on one part of the body can spread to other parts and eruptions will appear in one place and then another and then another. The rash can last from ten days to about three weeks although it can be longer in sensitive people.

Symptoms consist of blistery eruptions, redness, heat and great itching. The skin can swell, becoming very painful and it can affect all parts of the body. It can be a tormenting condition for those who are sensitive. Conventional treatment begins with antihistamines and calamine and moves to systemic steroids, either tablets or injections if very serious. Even then, it can take a while for real relief to settle in.

● HOMEOPATHIC CARE

If it is suspected that infection with poison oak or ivy has taken place, the first remedy to take is homeopathic poison ivy – *Rhus tox.* It is best to take one tablet three times daily for three days. If symptoms develop, continue this remedy to see if it helps. If it doesn't, a combination strategy should be employed, taking the following remedies: *Anacardium, Arsenicum album* and *Croton tiglium.* One tablet of each should be mixed in water and one tsp. taken four times daily for three to five days. Also *Rhus diversoloba* (another remedy from the same botanical family) can be tried if *Rhus tox* doesn't work or in combination with it in the beginning.

NOTE This is not easy to treat and there may be other indicated remedies. Professional homeopathic advice is recommended if relief is not found.

Scabies

Scabies is a common skin affection due to the scabies mite, a parasite that bores into the skin, causing immense itchiness. It is difficult to see but often one may see little black points or lines between the fingers or in the creases of the skin. Itching is often much worse at night and from the heat. It is highly infectious and easily caught by contact with others or by using the same bedding. The skin may blister or form small itchy lumps in various parts of the body. If one person has it, the whole family should be treated.

● GENERAL CARE

All clothing and bedding must be thoroughly washed and repeated even daily for one week. The mites are very tenacious. You can take one cup of kerosene/paraffin and mix with one cup of vegetable oil and apply twice daily for two days after washing, to all areas affected. Neem oil can also be used.

◗ HOMEOPATHIC CARE

Sulphur is a specific remedy for this condition and should be taken three times a day for up to seven days. Stop the remedy if relief of the itching is felt or if the itching gets much worse after the remedy. Other remedies may be indicated, including *Arsenicum album* if there is burning of the skin with great restlessness and anxiety. If the condition remains persistent, consider giving *Psorinum* for up to five days. It is a nosode made from scabies.

◢ HERBAL CARE

Use tea tree oil or lavender on the itchiest parts of the skin.

Shingles (Herpes Zoster)

Shingles is a viral condition affecting the skin and is connected to the chicken pox virus. It creates extremely painful swelling and blisters, irritating superficial nerves near the skin. It can affect any part of the body, including the face and also the torso and tends to often occur in one particular place. It most prominently affects elderly people and those under severe stress or suffering other immune compromised diseases such as AIDS. At times, the pain is the first symptom to occur before the rash appears. If untreated, it can last for weeks. Also, even after treatment, some people experience post herpetic neuralgia where areas of the skin remain inflamed. Conventional treatment involves pain relief and anti-viral drugs but it is not always that effective. However, it is important to give some pain relief medicine when it is very intense.

● HOMEOPATHIC CARE

Rhus tox is the first remedy to consider for shingles. It has the classic eruption of blisters (vesicles) which are burning, itching and with sharp stitching pains. The skin can look and feel thick. The eruptions may be dry, crusty and moist. The pains can be better for warm applications and if bad, you can feel chilled, as if cold water is being thrown over you. If that remedy doesn't work then *Mezereum* can be given, especially if it affects one side of the face only. The blisters may ooze sticky moisture and then form thick crusts. You may feel symptoms are better in the cool, open air. If the pains are very extreme, with shooting, stitching pains which can even make you cry, then *Ranunculus bulbosa* can be given. Eruptions may be especially on the chest, making it difficult to breathe and become much worse from any touch.

NOTE Skin conditions are not always easy to treat homeopathically. Finding the exact picture can be difficult. If *Rhus tox* doesn't work, then go to one of the other remedies or combine them both. If the pain is severe, then one should expect some relief in the pain within twelve hours to one day but it will take some days before new eruptions stop coming. Keep giving the remedy until significant relief is achieved. If there is some improvement over one week but then no further improvement is seen, give *Graphites*, one tablet four times a day for three to five days. *Mercurius* can also be considered if the eruptions are very painful and itch at night and *Arsenicum album* if there is despair from pain. Also, professional medical care may be needed, especially in elderly people and where the eyes are affected.

Ulcers

Skin ulcers are common in tropical climates and most commonly affect people below the knee, especially around the foot if the foot is mostly exposed through wearing flip-flops all the time. It often begins from a minor injury to the skin, when the skin is broken, even from scratching a bite or pimple and a secondary bacterial infection takes place. Gradually or at times quite suddenly the ulcer spreads and can become painful, and an offensive or watery discharge can be seen. Often these ulcers will eventually resolve but it is imperative to take good care of the wound to aid the healing and prevent complication. More serious complications involve infection of the bone, or a more systemic blood infection affecting the whole body and the development of much fibrous scar tissue, preventing healing. Therefore, especially when traveling, it is imperative to look after the wound, keep it clean and if very bad, to stop traveling until some healing has taken place. Ulcers can also come from a staphylococcal bacterial infection in the blood, and this can lead to recurrent ulcers on the skin, beginning as a small boil and quickly spreading into a large ulcer. They can take a long time to heal. One needs to be careful with a staphylococcal infection that it does not lead to a more general septic condition of the body. Medical intervention can be necessary.

● **GENERAL CARE**

An ulcer should be kept clean. It should be washed with clean, disinfected water, with some drops of *Calendula* lotion in a ratio of 1:10 approximately. Conventional antiseptic like hydrogen peroxide is also good. Any dead skin should be removed. If the wound is relatively superficial without pus formation, an oil based *Calendula* lotion can be used on the ulcer and then covered with a non-adhesive dressing or gauze. It is important that the dressing does not stick to the ulcer, which would prevent new skin from forming when the dressing is removed.

If the ulcer is deeper and there is pus formation, then *Calendula* solution should be mixed with some water (ratio of 1:10) and a dressing soaked in this solution should be put onto the ulcer. The dressing should always be wet and the *Calendula* mixture can be sprayed onto the dressing to keep it moist. Change the dressing daily. Clear plastic or a plastic bag can be used to cover the dressing to keep it moist. This should be continued until the infection is clean. If *Calendula* is not available use other local antiseptic lotions, such as hydrogen peroxide, isopropyl alcohol or iodine initially. These have also been counter indicated in superficial wounds due to their tendency to increase scar tissue and healing time. The most important thing is to initially clean the wound, using these or other products. Once the ulcer is clean, try and leave it exposed to the air, using only a small amount of calendula cream. If on the foot or lower leg, do not walk anymore than absolutely necessary. However if there is a need to travel the ulcer should be bandaged as described above.

Manuka honey or other honey is a strong antibacterial to treat ulcers and also burns. It can be used alongside *Calendula* to help heal the ulcer at both the initial stage of pus formation and for secondary healing. Tea tree oil can be used similarly.

● HOMEOPATHIC CARE

Arsenicum album is needed for ulcers with great burning but which may feel better from warm application. There can be anxiety and restlessness with the ulcer and it is for infected ulcers with offensive, burning discharges. *Carbo veg* is indicated for ulcers that are burning but which also can feel cold, and it is good for infected ulcers in which the skin is blue. *Lachesis* is needed for infected ulcers with a bluish/purple color and which are very sensitive to touch. The ulcer looks as though it is becoming very infected. It is the first remedy to think of ulcers which come from a bite of a poisonous animal. *Mercurius* is for ulcers with ragged edges with an offensive yellow discharge, which bleeds easily and the margins look like raw meat.

COMBINATION STRATEGY If in doubt, combine one tablet of *Mercurius*, *Arsenicum album*, *Carbo veg* and *Lachesis* in a glass of water and take one tsp. four times a day for three to five days.

Chapter Thirteen
Common Tropical Conditions

Disease Risks for Travelers
Prevention and Treatment

DENGUE FEVER Medium Risk

- Endemic in Sub-Saharan Africa, South East Asia, India, the Caribbean and Central and South America. Found more in urban areas
- A viral infection caught from mosquitoes.
- Avoiding being bitten by mosquitoes. Use of repellants, nets and clothing. Conventional treatment not available

MALARIA High Risk

- Endemic in all tropical areas, especially Sub-Saharan Africa, South East Asia and Amazonia of South America
- A parasitic infection caught from mosquitoes.
- Avoiding being bitten by mosquitoes. Use of conventional malaria prophylactics. Conventional treatment is available

---

Dengue Fever

ONSET Symptoms develop between 2-14 days from infection.
KEY SYMPTOMS Sudden onset of fever, aching and crippling bone and joint pains. Severe headache. It looks similar to malaria.

Dengue fever is a viral infection spread through mosquito bites. These mosquitoes are often found near human habitation and therefore dengue often occurs in more urban areas. It is found predominantly in Africa, South-East Asia, parts of South America, including the North East of Brazil and also in the Caribbean. Incubation of dengue can be anything between two days to two weeks, averaging around one week. In a majority of cases, there is a sudden onset of symptoms with a high fever and intense, crippling pain in the joints, bones and muscles. The sensation is often one of the bones feeling broken. There can be severe headache and fever which can last for some days. There can be a skin eruption with red patches. In most cases, there is a gradual remission and spontaneous recovery after the intense symptoms have abated but it can take some time. Homeopathy can be important here to help recovery. However, a more serious disease, dengue hemorrhagic fever may occur which can be fatal and needs professional care. There is no effective conventional treatment for dengue fever as it is a viral condition.
Also see Chapter Seven: Common Infections, Fever and Influenza

In the initial stages of the condition, it may seem like any other fever and you may likely need *Aconite*, *Belladonna* or *Bryonia*. Each remedy is useful when there is a high fever, which is often dry and burning.

However, the first remedy to think of in dengue is *Eupatorium perfoliatum*, as it has the characteristic bone breaking pains that are often seen. These pains are felt all over, but especially in the back. There can be an intense headache, fever, chill and often nausea and vomiting. The chill is often felt going up and down the back. *Gelsemium* can also look like *Eupatorium*, with aching in the joints and muscles and a chill in the back. However it often has more drowsiness, dullness and weakness and not the pain in the bones so strongly. *Rhus tox* also has great aching in the body but with much more restlessness. With the fever, there can be great chill, which is much worse from any uncovering. It can feel as if cold water is being poured over you.

It may occur that you give one remedy at the beginning of treatment and then need to move to another remedy as the picture changes. One needs to notice the shift in the symptom picture over a number of days. *Aconite* and *Belladonna* may often be indicated at the beginning and the other remedies later. *Bryonia* and *Rhus tox* can often be alternated as the symptom picture changes.

COMBINATION STRATEGY One can combine more than one remedy together, if a clear image is not seen. Choose between the remedies listed. *Eupatorium perfoliatum* however is the most likely remedy to be indicated in this condition.

Malaria

ONSET Symptoms come within 7-14 days of infection.
KEY SYMPTOMS Fever, chill, aching, weakness, sweating. Fever worse at night often, but can feel OK in the day. Periodical fevers, coming every 3-4 days. Great weakness. Diarrhea, which may be the first symptom seen. In children especially great anemia, with swelling of liver and spleen. Complications of meningitis – convulsions, coma, death.

Malaria is the biggest killer of any disease facing the planet, greater than AIDS and TB combined. For a traveler to Africa or parts of Asia, it is the most important disease to protect against. Conventionally, a variety of medications can be taken as a preventative against the disease. See Chapter Sixteen: Prevention, Malaria. Over the years, the recommended medications have changed as the disease has adapted and developed resistance against anti-malaria medications.

For short term travel to very risky parts of the world like Sub Saharan Africa and South East Asia, taking conventional anti-malarials makes sense, but it is important to find one that works for you and to evaluate the risks. Prevention is always the key. For travelers or others who are living in malaria areas for prolonged periods of time (six months or more), taking medication on a long term basis is not so realistic as the longer the medications are taken, the more possible are side effects. However, this is a very individual issue. Some people do fine on them, others do not. There is also a lack of research on the long term effects of anti-malarial medication and so drug companies are not able to make formal recommendations on their use. Also, drugs used to treat malaria can be less effective if medication has been taken for prevention. However, if you do choose to take anti-malarials for more than six months in a row, it is important to find the right drug to take, which is effective, affordable and with minimal side effects. Doxycyclin (an antibiotic) and Mefloquine (Larium) are two of the most common recommended, but each has its side effects, especially if taken for prolonged periods. Also, evaluation of the risks in different areas of a country or countries may allow for a relatively risk free gap in taking medication. However, most 'ex pats' living in tropical areas for prolonged periods do not take anti-malarials as a routine treatment. However, they often have immediate access to appropriate malarial treatment. If you are traveling for prolonged periods in a high risk malaria area and are not going to be near medical care, it is good to take some malaria medication with you in case of an attack. Many long- term 'ex pats' do get bouts of malaria from time to time. Basically, the longer one lives in a malaria country, the more likely one is to get a bout, sooner or later. Over time, most people living in a malarial country do acquire some immunity, depending on general health factors, but once leaving that country, the immunity does not last that long (6 months or so) and on returning, there is an increased risk again. Therefore, it is important to consider what other options there are to both protect and treat malaria. Natural medicines can be used in conjunction with conventional medication or on their own if it seems appropriate.

For shorter trips to malarial countries, the most important issues to consider are evaluating the risks of malaria where you are going and finding the appropriate anti-malarial if you choose to take them. More information on this is given below and much information is available on government and health websites.

Conventional medical channels and government bodies will not recommend most natural treatments, including homeopathy because of the lack of scientific proof that it works. However, in my experience working in Africa and seeing how local homeopaths are able to treat malaria, as well as growing evidence of homeopathy's prophylactic effect, I feel it is useful to have this information and use it, either in conjunction with conventional protocols or on their own if you choose. It is important you do the research and choose a strategy that works for you. *See Chapter Eighteen, Resources and References*

There are two basic forms of malaria. Most common is 'benign malaria' and can show as recurrent intermittent fevers (described often as tertian and quartian malaria) and other associated symptoms. For many living in malarial areas, they may get a new infection once to three times a year, with mild to serious symptoms but which can be treated fairly easily. There will be no attacks in between. The number of infections and seriousness of the attacks depends much on the constitution and basic susceptibility of a person. More serious is 'malignant malaria' in which the liver and spleen can be deeply and quickly affected leading to profound anemia and liver dysfunction. This type of malaria can often be fatal. There is often a lack of the periodicity found in the benign malaria but jaundice, anemia and other serious symptoms are seen in acute phases. Cerebral malaria is one of these conditions and leads to coma, convulsions and possible death. This has to be treated immediately. It is most lethal in young children and those with already weak immune systems. However, in more remote parts of Africa, many people simply have no access to any form of medical care and the largest mortality rates are amongst young malnourished children who cannot access health care of any kind.

Also, for many people in Africa and other endemic countries, there is a form of chronic (benign) malaria, which while not lethal, can generally undermine a person's health. Some people have it worse than others, but it also depends very much on overall immunity and the history of other conditions such as AIDS, T.B., malnutrition, etc. These forms of malaria are quite accessible to natural medicine. Visitors to countries who do get malaria can also experience recurrent bouts of malaria, even after returning to their home country and without subsequent re-infection. This can be treated with the same remedies listed below or with more constitutional homeopathic care.

It is also common for a person living in malaria areas to test positive for malaria yet have no symptoms and then get symptoms when unrelated events occur, such as physical or emotional stress. This can activate the condition as the liver can carry the parasite which then gets released due to stress. Correspondingly, during the first outbreak of symptoms, there can be at times no evidence of infection in the blood work. The incubation period can be up to two weeks from infection and the first bout of symptoms often lasts up to one week. The initial fever may last a few hours but after about eight hours, the temperature can be normal. However, within 3 days, another episode can begin (hence the term tertian malaria). Further attacks can occur over weeks until gradually they disappear. However, residual weakness, weight loss and swelling of the spleen and/or liver are quite common. For some people, that will be the end of attacks whereas for others, another bout can occur a few weeks later and after a number of episodes will again disappear until a new episode occurs weeks or months later. A less common type of malaria is called quartian malaria in that attacks occur every 4 days. This form tends to be stronger and more serious than the tertian attacks, with episodes occurring even years later.

There are various strains of malaria, the most dangerous one being Falciparum malaria. This relates to the particular parasitic infection. It is this strain which can cause the cerebral form of malaria that tends to kill young children so easily. It is important to know which type of malaria a person has in order to find the correct conventional treatment. This virulent form is often found in Sub-Saharan Africa, in particular West Africa.

◆ HOMEOPATHIC CARE

Treating malaria can be difficult using traditional homeopathic methodology, especially if one is treating oneself. It is highly recommended to get more professional care if at all possible. As mentioned, homeopathic treatment can be given in conjunction with conventional therapy. The following remedies are the most commonly used homeopathic remedies. The basic care for prevention can also be given at the same time as it is often the same treatment. See Chapter Sixteen: Prevention. Also study the main fever and influenza remedies in Chapter Seven: Common Infections, as in the acute phase, any remedy may be needed, especially *Aconite*, *Arsenicum album*, *Belladonna*, *Eupatorium perfoliatum*, *Ipecac* and *Nux vomica*.

Acute 1st phase (Benign and Malignant)

At this stage, it may not be clear that it is malaria. It can look like many other diseases, including dengue, influenza, Lassa fever, sunstroke, typhoid etc., and it is important to get tested. However, homeopathic remedies can be given, simply based on the symptom picture. For people who have already had a bout of malaria before, it is more obvious that it is a recurrence. Often there is a relatively sudden onset of fever, with periods of chill, alternating with heat and sweating. There may be extreme shivering in the chill phase. There is often weakness, a lack of appetite and at times diarrhea and vomiting. When experiencing fever or chill, you must stay hydrated. Take oral rehydration as that will help deal with the fever and consequent weakness. Water alone may not be sufficient to replenish fluids.

Arsenicum album is one of the first remedies to consider. There is fever, great shaking chill and a need to be covered. There can be intense nausea, vomiting and at times diarrhea. There is great weakness and restlessness and during the fever often a thirst for sips of water. In this stage the remedy needs to be given frequently, one tsp. every ten to fifteen minutes in water. *Nux vomica* is also often indicated and is similar to *Arsenicum album*. There is pain in the abdomen, often with violent intense vomiting and urging for stool. There can be pains in the liver and spleen which is much worse from any touch to the region. *Belladonna* is needed when sudden, intense, very hot and dry fever is seen.

Eupatorium perfoliatum is a good remedy when there are intense aching pains in the bones, feeling as if they would break. This is throughout the body, including the back. There can be great nausea and vomiting, often of bile and great, shaking chill. *Ipecac* has intense nausea and vomiting in all stages, along with a fever. There can be a great sinking feeling in the stomach. There may be no thirst, even in heat, but often can have a clean tongue.

China may also be needed in the acute stage when there is a marked periodicity to symptoms but more often is indicated when there is an ongoing recurrence of symptoms or in particularly intense bouts of malaria when the liver and spleen are swollen.

See malignant malaria below and Chapter Seven: Common Infections, Fever section

COMBINATION STRATEGY If the picture is not clear, put one tablet of all the remedies above in a glass and take a sip (one tsp.) every ten to fifteen minutes for four hours and then once hourly after this. Look for some relief in four hours to one day but it will take longer to see serious improvement. As mentioned, it is hard to find the exact remedy so combining all the remedies ensures that ideally one of them will work.

Chronic recurrence (Benign)

China is needed when there is a fever that comes in exact phases and there can be great ringing in the ears. There is great fatigue and often abdominal fullness and pain and swelling in the liver area. In the fever stage, there can be drenching sweats which are exhausting. There can be great abdominal bloating, a lack of appetite and diarrhea. (Also to be considered are *Chinium arsenicosum* – when nausea and vomiting and extreme weakness are felt and *Chinium sulphuricum* – when dizziness and tinnitus predominate and also exact periodicity of complaints).

Natrum muriaticum is given in more chronic conditions when there is an intense, splitting headache, weakness, perspiration, great thirst and fever that comes in marked phases. *Sulphur* needs to be given if other remedies have been given and do not work fully and you feel just exhausted and flat, but without any other clear symptoms.

Baptisia and *Pyrogen* can also be given when the malaria fever has become totally exhausting and you feel simply exhausted and prostrated, with fever and aching, and a bruised soreness over the whole body.

See Chapter Seven: Common Infections, Influenza section

NOTE These remedies can also be indicated in the acute first phase and especially *China* can be combined with other remedies in the first phases of malaria. Even if you are taking conventional medication for malaria, you can still take some homeopathic remedies to help. Or after finishing medication you can see what symptoms are remaining and give a remedy. If in doubt, simply take *China* 30c, twice daily for one week to aid recovery.

Malignant Malaria

Often the liver and spleen are affected (and also with benign malaria), and profound anemia is seen. This needs to be treated by a medical expert and conventional therapy given. Homeopathic remedies can be used alongside as necessary. *Ceanothus* is a specific remedy for swelling of the liver and spleen with anemia. It should ideally be given in a low potency, e.g., 6c and repeated frequently for one to two weeks. *China* has swelling of the liver and of the whole abdomen. There is jaundice and anemia with great bloating and little appetite. There is great weakness. *Chinium arsenicosum* is also a useful remedy when there is profound weakness, anemia, nausea and vomiting. These remedies can be given in a 6c or 30c potency and repeated 3 times daily for at least one week.

⬥ HERBAL CARE

These are more effective in the acute and chronic relapse phases. Neem tincture (Azadrachita indica – Margosa bark), Artemisia annua (Sweet wormwood), Eucalyptus (in a tincture from the leaves and/or in a homeopathic potency up to 6x or 6c).

These should be given up to ten times a day in tincture, five drops each time. They can be taken along with homeopathic remedies. Neem and artemesia can also be taken in a tea form (5-10 grams of dried leaf, 1tr of boiling water poured over them and drunk slowly through the day. Make separately. Use less for children. 10 grams is used in more serious cases. Pregnant women should not use this, especially in first trimester). Knowing a good source of neem and artemesia is useful and both are widely found in the tropics. Lemon grass tea should be taken for any fever, 1-2 liters daily.

See Chapter Sixteen: Prevention

Typhoid

ONSET Incubation is between 7-10 days. Easily confused with malaria in early stages.

KEY SYMPTOMS Fever resembling influenza, sore throat, abdominal pains. Fever coming and going. High fever in children with diarrhea, vomiting. After 1-2 weeks, diarrhea becomes worse, great weakness, fever becomes more debilitating with weakness and delirium. Lung symptoms with bloody mucus with cough. Bloody stools, leading to perforation of the bowels.

Typhoid is a bacterial infection and is one of the most serious and common conditions in the tropical regions of the world. For travelers, the Indian subcontinent, Sub Saharan Africa and Latin America carry the most risk. It is caught from food or water contaminated with Salmonella bacteria. The incubation period for typhoid is around ten days, but can be less than that, as well as much longer (which should be considered if one gets sick even weeks after returning home). Even though there are characteristic symptoms of the disease as it develops, in many cases the disease can go unnoticed until serious symptoms develop. Often it looks similar to influenza, with a general unwell feeling, fever, sore throat, cough and generalized abdominal pains. One of the most characteristic qualities about typhoid is that the pulse can remain unusually low even though the temperature is rising. This is one of the most important things to notice if typhoid is suspected. However, in many cases, this may not be seen but typhoid always needs to be considered in such situations and a test can be done, especially to differentiate from malaria as it is not uncommon to see a fever come and go in apparent phases. (At this point the homeopathic remedy may not be obvious but pay careful attention to the symptoms). Symptoms in children may be serious, with high fever, diarrhea and vomiting and also with a stiff neck, resembling meningitis. There may even be convulsions.

At the beginning, there may simply be some loose stools. Then after one to two weeks, a fever begins and there can be constipation at this point, and often a generalized body pain and headache. As the symptoms develop into the second week there are more distinct abdominal symptoms with sensitivity around the appendix area and the liver and spleen become swollen. Symptoms can get worse into the third week, with diarrhea developing and great weakness, confusion, disorientation and even delirium. There can be a severe headache, especially felt in the neck area. If untreated, this can last weeks, with symptoms changing but no real recovery. There can be intestinal bleeding even leading to perforation of the bowel. Other complications of typhoid include pneumonia, inflammation of the heart, acute arthritis, abscess of the spleen and other conditions. Gradually recovery will take place if there are not serious complications.

Because of the difficulty in diagnosis, it is important that treatment is begun as soon as possible. Conventional treatment can be effective in these cases, including the need for blood transfusions, and rehydration. However, homeopathic treatment can also be given alongside any conventional treatment and can greatly help the body recover from this disease. The earlier homeopathic and conventional treatment is given, the better the prognosis. However, a clear picture for a homeopathic remedy is not always obvious in the beginning. Try and wait until the picture becomes clear.

Even after recovery, some people still excrete the typhoid bacteria in the feces and urine for a number of months. Therefore, these people can spread the disease unbeknownst to themselves and others. It is also important that the patient is well looked after during the period of recovery, with simple, clean food, juices and water. Heavy food, dairy and meat should be avoided. Recovery can be quite slow.

See Chapter Six: Digestive Conditions, Diarrhea and Dysentery and Chapter Seven: Common Infections, Fever and Influenza

● HOMEOPATHIC CARE

Nearly all the important remedies needed are described in Chapter Seven: Common Infections, Fever and Influenza. However, it is important to know the differences between the remedies as well as to have a diagnosis of the condition. One can give homeopathic remedies even when conventional treatment is given.

In the beginning stages, *Arsenicum album* is often indicated and the most important symptoms are weakness, chill, restlessness and anxiety. *Rhus tox* is indicated when there is great aching and restlessness. There is often a great chill and desire to be covered and the body feels as if dashed with water. There is a chill in single parts of the body. The aching is intense, with rheumatic type symptoms, which can be stitching, tearing and shooting, with great restlessness.

Baptisia is the first remedy to consider once you really know it is typhoid and/or when it is in the second stage of the condition. There is great prostration, with weakness and aching of muscles. You can't get comfortable, and the bed feels hard. There is a dullness and confusion in the mind. Parts of your body feel scattered over the bed or as if your body is in pieces. You fall asleep when answering questions in a passive type of delirium. Your face often looks dusky, besotted and stupid. The fever is low but you feel as if you are sinking into the bed and there is an offensive odor from the body.

Bryonia and *Gelsemium* have to be compared with *Baptisia*, in both the first and second stage of typhoid. *Bryonia* has symptoms of a fever with delirium. You want to be quiet and be left alone. In a delirium, you can say you want to go home, even though there. Pains are worse from any motion or jar. You can have a great headache, as if your head is splitting open and it becomes worse from any motion or coughing. Joints can be inflamed and swollen and there is soreness in the abdomen, which is worse from pressure. *Gelsemium* has symptoms of weakness, heaviness, soreness and sleepiness. Your eyelids look very heavy and the face sleepy.

You have a low state of fever with a severe headache, especially in the back of the head, (occipital). Mentally, there is dullness, confusion and often dizziness. With fever, there is often chill, with great aching and chill is found going up and down the back. Often there is a lack of thirst during the heat phase of fever.

Ipecac is indicated when there is great nausea and respiratory symptoms with cough and bleeding from the lungs. There can be a profuse nose bleeding with cough and other symptoms. The cough is suffocating and there is rattling in the chest without expectoration. *Ipecac* is indicated more in the second stage of typhoid. *Phosphorus* also has similar respiratory symptoms with coughing and bleeding from the lungs and with nosebleed. The cough is often hacking and dry, with a great tightness around the chest. Ideally at this stage you will have professional medical help.

Muriatic acidum is indicated in more serious typhoid cases, with great prostration and aching of muscles. Mucous membranes of the mouth are dry, bleeding, cracked and ulcerated and the face is dark red. There is great soreness of the body causing restlessness. There is muttering with loud moaning and there can be intense burning heat with aversion to covers. It will often be compared with *Baptisia* and also *Pyrogen*. *Pyrogen* is indicated in the second stage, when the fever becomes 'septic', and you feel an intense, bruised soreness, with bone pains and the odor of the body and breath is foul. The pulse is either very quick or very slow. With a fever, there can be excitability, loquacity or great confusion, and like with *Baptisia*, a sense of duality in the body. Chills are often felt between the shoulder blades. It is given when other remedies have not worked well and you are sinking lower into the disease. Hopefully medical help will be available in such circumstances.

COMBINATION STRATEGY Given the complexity of the disease and the difficulty finding the correct homeopathic remedy, one can mix together a number of remedies to cover the situation. However, if a picture is clear, then give the single remedy first. This is the best way to approach this. But if necessary, mix together *Arsenicum album*, *Baptisia*, *Bryonia*, *Gelsemium* and *Rhus tox* if aching and low mental states are dominant, even with delirium. If hemorrhage is seen, then mix together

Ipecac and *Phosphorus*. If low, septic states predominate, mix together *Baptisia*, *Muriatic acid* and *Pyrogen*. Improvement may be slow but some signs should be seen in one to two days. The remedy should be repeated in water, one tsp. every one to two hours when it is severe and only reduced when symptoms improve. It should still be given two to three times a day for at least one week.

If a single remedy is given and the picture changes stop the remedy and consider a new remedy. Do not wait too long. Another remedy should be found if there is a change of symptoms. However, if a remedy is working, do not change it. Continue until a new picture emerges. In typhoid, recovery is slow, even with the correct remedy.

🌿 HERBAL CARE

Take eucalyptus tincture – and/or homeopathic dose of 6x or 6c. It should be taken three to four times a day at the beginning of any symptoms. *Echinacea* tincture can also be taken.

Chapter Fourteen

Other Tropical And Infectious Conditions

Most of these diseases are extremely rare for most travelers. Of the diseases described, Bilharzia is the most common and serious condition seen. However, other diseases are mentioned as they are endemic to certain regions of the world often traveled in and also where preventative methods can be taken.

For most of these diseases if homeopathic treatment is suitable, remedies are recommended or are referred to other relevant chapters, especially Chapter Seven: Common Infections as fevers are a common aspect of many of these diseases.

Disease Risks for Travelers
Prevention and Treatment

AFRICAN SLEEPING SICKNESS (HUMAN AFRICAN TRYPANOSOMIASIS) Fairly Low Risk

- Found in Sub-Saharan Africa (West, Central and East Africa)
- Parasite spread by tsetse fly. In West Africa, found mainly

---

around rivers and water. In East Africa, found around drier bush land

- Prevent being bitten. Using insect repellants is important. Conventional treatment is available

BILHARZIA (SCHISTOSOMIASIS) High Risk

- Endemic throughout the world. Especially seen in Sub-Saharan Africa, The Nile region of Egypt, South America, The Caribbean, China, Philippines and Japan
- A worm which infects an aquatic snail found in fresh water areas and spreads to humans. All fresh water, e.g., lakes, rivers, streams is suspect
- If in fresh water, wear clothes or boots, wet suits etc. Rub off well if getting wet. Be careful swimming in lakes. Check out disease incidence. Conventional treatment is available

BRUCELLOSIS Low Risk

- Endemic throughout the world, but not that common.
- Bacteria spread from unpasteurized milk products. More likely seen in countries that use unpasteurized milk, especially goat products
- Only eat and drink pasteurized products or where the manufacture of raw products is extremely hygienic. Conventional treatment is available

CHAGAS DISEASE (AMERICAN TRYPTOMANIASIS) Low Risk

- Found mostly in rural areas of Central and South America
- A parasite spread through the bite of an insect.
- Be careful if staying in homes of poor people in rural areas. Conventional treatment works well in acute phase, less well in chronic phases

CHOLERA Low Risk

- Endemic in areas of extremely poor hygiene and trauma due to war. More seen in Africa, the Indian subcontinent and South East Asia
- A bacterial infection spread through contaminated food and water
- Avoid areas of epidemic if possible and ensure food and water is clean. Conventional treatment is effective if done early.
- Vaccine available but only 50-60% effective

DIPHTHERIA Low Risk

- Found now occasionally in developing countries, but as widely vaccinated against, it is not common. Rare outbreaks in developed nations
- A bacterial infection spread from person to person via the nose and mouth.
- Avoid contact with any infected people, even if unsure of diagnosis. Conventional treatment is effective, but it can be serious if complicated and in small children

FILIARIASIS Low Risk

- Found in tropical areas of the world, especially Asia, Africa and South and Central America
- A roundworm infection, spread through black flies and mosquitoes. One form of disease leads to Elephantiasis
- Avoid being bitten by mosquitoes using repellants, nets etc.
- Conventional treatment is effective

GUINEA WORM (DRACUNUCULIASIS) Low Risk

- Found in India, West and Central Africa, South America, but now mostly in Sub-Saharan Africa, and mainly in South Sudan

- A worm infection spread from fleas
- Avoid drinking stagnant water. Be aware of skin infections, developing ulcers. There is no conventional treatment but secondary infections can be treated

HOOKWORM DISEASE Low Risk (If care Is taken)

- Endemic throughout the world, especially Sub-Saharan Africa, South and Central America and Asia. One of the most insidious and common diseases of tropical areas, especially for children
- A worm infection, the larvae penetrating the feet when walking barefoot. Not normally fatal but contributes to chronic health problems, especially in children
- Avoid walking barefoot, especially where any fecal matter is present. Feces used as fertilizer increases risk as is any poor hygiene. Wash hands frequently. More found in sandy, loamy soil. Conventional treatment is available

JAPANESE ENCEPHALITIS Low Risk

- Found mainly throughout Asia, predominantly in rural areas and during summer, fall and monsoon time
- A viral infection spread via mosquitoes
- Avoid being bitten by mosquitoes. Be careful if in rural areas of flood, irrigation and in summer months

LASSA FEVER Low Risk

- Found mainly in West Africa in rural areas
- A virus spread through food contaminated with infected mouse and rats' urine, e.g., stored grain reserves. Also can be caught through respiratory tract. Very serious disease
- Avoid eating food that could be contaminated. As found mainly in rural areas, knowing the incidence of the disease is useful. Avoid contact with anybody with the disease. Conventional treatment somewhat effective

LEISHMANIASIS Low Risk

- Endemic in Sub-Saharan Africa, India, China, Central and South America and Southern Europe. Often found in urban areas
- A parasitic disease spread through the bites of sand flies, dogs often being the carriers of the disease. A serious disease with many complications
- If in areas of infection, use repellants, similar as for mosquitoes. A finer net is needed than for mosquitoes. Conventional treatment is effective

LEPTOSPIROSIS Low Risk

- Endemic in South East Asia and parts of Cuba but also found in other warm climates
- A bacterial disease spread through contact with water contaminated with infected rats and mice urine
- If in areas during monsoons and floods where the disease occurs, avoid contact with water, especially if skin is broken. Conventional treatment is effective

PLAGUE Low Risk

- Only found fairly rarely today in developing countries, e.g., India. Historically it devastated Europe in the 1300's
- A bacterial infection spread by fleas carried by rodents. Historically a very serious disease with very high fatality
- Only Naturalists are normally at risk. However, avoid sleeping and living in dirty places where rats have been. A vaccine is available. Conventional treatment is effective

POLIOMYELITIS Low Risk

- Rarely seen today because of widespread vaccination, it still occurs in developing countries such as India, South East Asia, the Middle East and Africa

- A viral disease caught through inhalation, from direct contact with infected mucus, phlegm or feces. Mostly not serious but 1% develop forms of paralysis
- Avoid contact with infected people. Avoid contact with children in developing countries who were just given the 'live' vaccine

RABIES Low Risk

- Found in isolated incidences in developing countries. Rarely seen in developed countries
- A viral disease caught from saliva of infected animal, usually a dog, bat, fox, skunk, raccoon etc. A very serious disease, it is often fatal if symptoms develop
- Avoid contact with dogs and other animals in developing countries. Avoid contact with bats and wild animals in developed countries. Conventional treatment is effective if done early enough. A vaccination is available

RIFT VALLEY FEVER Low Risk

- Found in South and Eastern Africa
- A viral disease spread by mosquitoes
- Prevention of being bit by mosquitoes. A self limiting disease

RIVER BLINDNESS (ONCOCERCIASIS) Low Risk

- Endemic in Sub-Saharan Africa and pockets of Central and South America
- A parasitic disease transmitted through the bite of a black fly
- Avoid being bitten by flies. Wear appropriate clothing. Conventional treatment is available

TRACHOMA Low Risk

- Found in many developing countries
- Chronic bacterial infection, affecting people with poor nutrition and hygiene
- Avoid any infection to the eye and treat immediately if infection occurs. Hygiene is key. Conventional treatment is available

WEST NILE VIRUS Low Risk

- Found in all parts of the world, including Europe and the U.S.
- A viral disease spread via mosquitoes, also affects birds and animals.
- Avoid being bitten by mosquitoes. Elderly and immune compromised people more affected. Conventional treatment is available

YELLOW FEVER Low Risk

- Endemic in Africa and South and Central America. Widely vaccinated against and therefore not seen much
- A viral disease transmitted through mosquitoes. It can be serious with fatalities but most people recover
- Avoid being bitten by mosquitoes in tropical areas where the disease exists. There is no effective conventional treatment but supportive treatment can be given if serious

African Sleeping Sickness
(Human African Trypanosomiasis)

ONSET Symptoms can come on slowly. Initial symptoms may be absent and only months or years later will symptoms develop. Medical intervention is crucial.

KEY SYMPTOMS Fever. Head and body aches, coming and going. Swelling of lymph nodes. Neurological problems, tremors, convulsions, lack of coordination. Lethargy, sleepiness. Character change, argumentative, fitful, indifference.

This is known as sleeping sickness and is a parasitic disease spread by the tsetse fly. It is found mainly in rural areas of Sub-Saharan Africa and most prominent sleeping sickness cases are found in West, Central and East Africa. Over sixty million people are affected. In West Africa, the tsetse flies are found mainly around rivers and other watery areas. In East Africa, they are found more in drier bush land areas. Travelers are not that likely to come across this condition unless some time is spent in such areas. In urban areas, there is no real problem. Even in rural areas, infection rates vary widely in a similar geographical area. It is worth investigating this if time is to be spent in such areas. It can also be spread from mother to child, from blood transfusions and perhaps through sexual transmission.

The West and Central African variety can begin very slowly and without any noticeable symptoms for months and even years. However, within some weeks of infection, there may be symptoms of fever, headache, body aches etc., but which can come and go, with periods of well-being in between. There may be swelling of the liver and spleen and much swelling of lymph nodes in the body. There may develop more serious symptoms at this point and medical intervention is crucial. In some cases, these symptoms will be absent and the first real signs will be problems in the central nervous system, with problems walking, tremors, convulsions etc. The sleeping sickness symptoms are seen in this phase, often with great lethargy. Prior to this there may be some character changes, with fitful, argumentative behavior and indifference.

This may occur even years after initial infection, so if a person has spent any lengths of time in areas of infection and then suddenly develops behavioral or neurological conditions, this should be considered.

The East African variety tends to produce a more acute picture earlier on. Symptoms will include a local red, hot swelling around the area of the bite within days followed between one to three weeks later with symptoms of fever and lymphatic swellings described above. Again, medical diagnosis and treatment is crucial as it can lead to death within a number of weeks up to one year after infection. In the West African variety, death can occur over two to three years after initial infection.

● **GENERAL CARE**

Prevention of being bitten is important. Insect repellants should be used as needed and also pyrethrum spray can be used.
See Chapter Sixteen: Prevention, Malaria

◗ **HOMEOPATHIC CARE**

Professional care is ideally needed.
See Chapter Seven: Common Infections, Fever and Influenza

Bilharzia
(Schistosomiasis).

ONSET Nothing may be seen for up to two years from infection. There may be some initial skin irritation, but often nothing is noticed. In other cases, symptoms of fever, diarrhea, cough, skin irritation are seen within 8 weeks.
KEY SYMPTOMS Blood in urine. Inflammation of bladder, prostate and genitalia. Fever, malaise, diarrhea, skin rash, cough. Dysentery, blood and mucus in bowel. Liver and spleen enlarged.

Bilharzia is one of the most common serious diseases in certain regions of the world, predominantly Africa, South America and Asia. Only malaria has more impact on affected societies.

There are four or five varieties, each affecting different organs although the symptom pictures may be similar. It is an endemic condition throughout the world caused by a worm called Schistosomes which infect an aquatic snail found in fresh water areas. Once they leave the snail they infect the human host and from there, move to various organs of the body, causing acute and potentially serious chronic consequences. Therefore, the most important thing for the traveler is to avoid fresh water in those regions, including lakes, rivers and ponds, etc., any standing water in which snails may exist. It can be highly infectious and slight exposure to the water, like wading across a stream, may cause infection. Prevention is the best course. Do not swim in open fresh water, do not expose parts of the body to the water; avoid dammed water and if exposed, dry off and change clothes as quickly as possible. Do not stay wet and wear clothing or a wet suit to cross bodies of water.

One form of the disease affects the urinary organs, including the kidney, the prostate and the uterus. This form of bilharzia is found mainly in most of Africa and especially in the Nile region of Egypt. The incubation period after initial infection may take up to two years to manifest, making the initial diagnosis difficult. There may be some mild initial itching of the skin after infection, but little more. The first symptoms to be seen may be blood in the urine, especially at the end of urination, and then may develop into cystitis, kidney stones, prostate and uterine infection and even cancer of organs such as the bladder.

Other forms of the disease primarily affect the bowel and the liver. These forms are found in Africa and also in South America (especially the North East of Brazil), parts of the Caribbean, China, Japan and the Philippines. These forms may be more lethal than the first. Symptoms develop more quickly, up to eight weeks after infection, with the onset of a fever, general malaise, diarrhea, a generalized skin rash and cough. At this point, only a blood test will reveal the nature of the disease as it can look like many other conditions, especially malaria. After the fever goes, bowel symptoms can begin with dysentery, with blood and mucus in the stool. From there, the liver and spleen may become enlarged and kidney function begins to fail, leading to heart failure.

In another form of the disease, the initial skin condition may be very intense and the subsequent fever also very intense. There will also be blood in the stool and enlargement of the liver and spleen and there can be great hard swelling of the abdomen. There may be significant amounts of blood in the stool.

● HOMEOPATHIC CARE

This is best treated professionally and it is imperative that a diagnosis is made to confirm the cause of the symptoms. However, if one is traveling and self-treatment is necessary, the following remedies can be considered: *Antimonium tart* is good if there are symptoms of great weakness, breathlessness and profound drowsiness. The local bladder or other symptoms are less significant here but may be seen. *China* has great weakness, and also has abdominal symptoms such as bloating, lack of appetite and loose stools creating exhaustion. See Chapter Six: Digestive Conditions, Dysentery and Indigestion sections. There may be blood in the stool. *Terebinthina* is a specific remedy if the main symptom is bleeding from the bladder and also for great burning in the bladder, prostate and/or uterine area. It has abdominal bloating, dysentery and even colitis symptoms. Much bleeding is the key symptom along with burning.

Brucellosis

ONSET Symptoms are seen up to 3 to 4 weeks after infection. They may be mild or severe.
KEY SYMPTOMS Fever, chill, joint pains, testicular pain and swelling. Sweat with sour odor. Prolonged periodical fever. Weakness, swelling of liver and spleen.

This is a bacterial disease spread through drinking unpasteurized milk products. Symptoms develop up to three to four weeks after infection and can be either quite mild or more severe. The more severe symptoms include a high fever, often with chills, intense joint pains and also inflammation of the testicle, called orchitis or epididymitis. There may also be much sweating with a sour odor. The more chronic symptoms include a periodic fever in which the fever gradually gets worse over one week and then gradually comes back to normal over another week and then begins to rise again a few days later. This pattern can continue for months. There is also great weakness, with enlargement of the liver and spleen in some cases, ongoing perspiration and general exhaustion. The disease will eventually burn itself out in the vast majority of cases but can be treated effectively with homeopathy.

● HOMEOPATHIC CARE

Arsenicum album, *Baptisia*, *Bryonia*, *Eupatorium perfoliatum* and *Gelsemium* are most indicated. *Pulsatilla* is good when there is inflammation of the testes involved.

See Chapter Seven: Common Infections, Fever and Influenza sections

Chagas Disease
(American Trypanosomiasis)

ONSET Often very slow. Initial infection as a child and only as an adult do symptoms develop. In children, there may be a boil developing 1-4 weeks after bite. Then fever comes 1-2 weeks later.
KEY SYMPTOMS In children, they may have a bite, becoming a boil, lasting for months. Conjunctivitis, with swelling of lymph glands. Sudden, intense fever, lasting weeks, and swelling of liver and spleen. Inflammation of brain and heart. In adult, symptoms of heart disease, tendency to strokes, general weakness and digestive problems.

This is a parasitic infection due to the bite of an insect and is found in rural areas of Central and South America. It is a very common disease, found in both acute and long term chronic phases, affecting up to eleven million people, most of who don't know they are infected. Most urban travelers are unlikely to see this disease even though it is quite widespread throughout the region. For most people after infection, there is no apparent illness and the disease remains dormant for many years until the person is an adult in their twenties or thirties. If symptoms do appear in the initial phase and this is mostly with children, there may be skin sensitivity around the area of the bite, resembling a boil, which will last for months. If the point of infection is the eye, then a swelling of the upper and lower eyelids takes place with conjunctivitis and swelling of the lymph glands under the jaw on the affected side. (There is a tendency to bite the cheeks of the face, hence the term 'kissing bugs' is given to the insect. They are also called 'assassin bugs'). Around one week after this, a sudden and intense fever may arise and continue even for weeks. There can be further complications with swelling of the liver and spleen and in very severe cases, heart and brain inflammation, often leading to death. However, the majorities of people do survive this attack but are then prone to serious complications many years later, such as heart weakness, strokes, digestive problems and intellectual weakness.

● HOMEOPATHIC CARE

In the acute phase, a remedy must be chosen on the symptom picture. *Ledum*, one tablet three times daily for one week is an obvious one to begin for the affect of the bite, but other remedies for the fever must be considered. In the chronic phase, constitutional care must be sought, along with other medical options.
See Chapter Seven: Common Infections, Fever and Influenza sections

Cholera

ONSET Symptoms come on 2-7 days after infection with sudden attack of diarrhea.
KEY SYMPTOMS Sudden onset of violent diarrhea, very copious rice water and mostly painless. Intense vomiting, chill, cramping and spasms in intestines and throughout body.

Cholera is a bacterial disease and is spread through contaminated water and food. Certain people can be carriers of the disease and once infected, the incubation period is normally between two to seven days. Characteristically, there is a sudden onset of violent diarrhea, which becomes extremely copious, like rice water, and is painless. Often there is projectile vomiting, the great risk being a serious lack of fluids in the body, which if not replaced can lead to kidney failure and death. Therefore, the key to any treatment is rehydration. If possible this is done intravenously but if in remote areas and where no medical help is available, oral rehydration has to suffice. However, homeopathic medicines can be crucial to help the body recover and in cholera epidemics of the nineteenth century, homeopathy showed remarkable successes. In many cases, one may be infected by the cholera bacteria but show very mild symptoms which will not need much treatment.

See Chapter Five: Digestive Conditions, Diarrhea section

● HOMEOPATHIC CARE

The first remedy to consider is *Arsenicum album*. At this stage you may not even know it is cholera and often it will simply get better and you won't know it was a cholera infection. Not all cholera becomes life threatening and if you remain hydrated and are strong, it does not need to become serious. However, the symptoms you may feel will be nausea, vomiting and often diarrhea, all at the same time. There can be great weakness, restlessness and chilliness. *Veratrum album* may be needed if *Arsenicum album* doesn't work and if you have profuse cold perspiration on the forehead.

You can need *Camphor* if you feel a great icy coldness of the body yet you do not want to be covered and you can feel anxiety and even despair, along with some cramping. *Cuprum* should be taken if the cramping becomes really intense in any part of the body.

COMBINATION STRATEGY You can combine one or more of the remedies together in water and give one tsp. every hour until some relief.

Diphtheria

ONSET Symptoms appear 5-7 days after infection with sudden very sore throat. Symptoms often peak on the 4th day.
KEY SYMPTOMS Extreme sore throat, lymph glands of neck swollen and painful. Swelling in larynx, membrane forming in mouth, nose and throat, making breathing noisy. Offensive odor from mouth. Weakness but no fever.

This bacterial infection is rarely seen now, partly due to improvements in hygiene and partly due to it being part of the normal vaccination schedule for children. It may be seen while traveling in developing countries and any actual incidence of the condition should be treated with antibiotics. It is rarely seen in the developed world now. It is passed on via the oral route and incubates for up to five days. However, if it is found, symptoms will include a very sore throat, fever and headache. Lymph glands of the neck will be enlarged and painful, along with offensive breath. Breathing will become very noisy due to the swelling of the larynx and the formation of a membrane in the mouth, throat and nose. The membrane coating will be dark and the person gets weaker and quiet, but mostly has no fever. Conventional antibiotic therapy is effective for diphtheria.
See Chapter Nine: ENT, Throat Conditions and Chapter Seven: Common Infections

◆ HOMEOPATHIC CARE
Indicated homeopathic remedies include *Mercurius* and *Phytolacca* in particular and also *Lachesis* and *Rhus tox*.

Filiariasis

This is a disease of many tropical areas of the world and is a roundworm infection, which can eventually lead to elephantiasis, a fairly common affliction seen in India and Africa. The classic symptoms are gross swelling of the extremities and even the scrotum due to blocked lymphatic vessels. It may begin with painful inflammation of the lymph glands and/or testicles. Most ordinary travelers are at very low risk of catching this disease.

◐ HOMEOPATHIC CARE

This requires professional care, both homeopathic and conventional treatment.

Guinea Worm (Dracunuculiasis)

ONSET Symptoms are often seen only one year after infection.
KEY SYMPTOMS Skin itches, becomes red and burning, followed by a blistery eruption on skin, oozing a milky fluid, becoming an ulcer.

A water-born infection from drinking infected stagnant water which contains the larva of the worm that then infects the body, growing into worms which eventually make their way to the surface of the skin. The first symptoms seen, often one year after infection, are redness, itching and burning of the skin, with or without fever. The skin may break, creating a blister and a painful ulcer develops, which emits a milky fluid (larval worms). There can also be more serious complications such as blood poisoning, abscess formation and arthritis. This condition is found in India, West and Central Africa and Brazil and possibly other South American countries.

● GENERAL CARE

The ulcer needs to be kept clean to allow healing.
See Chapter Twelve: Skin Conditions, Ulcers section

◐ HOMEOPATHIC CARE

Silicea can be given to help the removal of the worm and larva, one tablet twice daily for one to two weeks.

Hookworm Disease

ONSET Often very few initial symptoms until more chronic conditions appear. Local itching on skin may be seen.
KEY SYMPTOMS Anemia in children, with weakness, fatigue and breathlessness. Intellectual and growth retardation in children. Digestive problems, nausea, vomiting, diarrhea.

This is a worm infestation that enters the body through the feet. They suck the blood of their host, which eventually leads to anemia, weakness, fatigue and breathlessness. Avoidance of walking barefoot is crucial as is replacement of iron and other nutrients from blood loss. They are found throughout Sub-Saharan Africa, the Americas and throughout Asia. In children, they cause intellectual and growth retardation and there is estimated to be between 500-600 million cases in the world. There may be local itching of the part infected by larvae but often no signs are seen until more chronic symptoms appear. This is why it is such a serious condition as there are few signs of infection and ways to treat it before it becomes more serious. Anemia is one of the most common signs of chronic infection, along with developmental issues in young children. In some cases there can be much digestive disturbance.

Do not walk barefoot in general, especially where there may be any fecal matter. They are found more in sandy and loamy soils than clay. Be aware even on beaches if people have been defecating nearby.

● HOMEOPATHIC CARE

Silicea can be given, as for Guinea worm, but professional care may be needed. Other symptomatic homeopathic treatment can be given.

Japanese Encephalitis

ONSET Symptoms appear 5-15 days after infection, mostly with sudden fever.

KEY SYMPTOMS Sudden fever, with headache and vomiting. Neurological symptoms, tremor, weakness, paralysis and stiff neck, with meningeal irritation.

Japanese encephalitis is a viral disease spread through mosquitoes. It is found in most parts of Asia, including the Indian Subcontinent, South East Asia and Far East Asia. It is found predominantly in rural, agricultural areas, often in times of flood, heavy rain, and around rice plantations. In more temperate parts of Asia, it occurs mainly in summer and fall, whereas in more tropical regions it occurs more with monsoons and due to irrigation practices. Children are much more affected in endemic areas. Most cases are asymptomatic but about 30,000-50,000 cases are reported annually. However, for travelers it is very low risk. Only 55 published reports of the disease were recorded from 1973 to 2008. It is estimated that in people from non-endemic countries there is less than one case per million travelers. However, for those who stay for prolonged periods of time in endemic regions where the disease exists, that rate will rise to that of the resident population. Most travelers though are at very low risk.

The incubation period is between five to fifteen days. Symptoms can develop suddenly with fever, headache and vomiting. Neurological disturbances may be seen, with weakness, tremor, stiff neck and meningeal irritation, rigidity of the body, paralysis, weakness and convulsions.

There is a vaccine for those especially at risk, but for most travelers, it is not necessary.

● **GENERAL CARE**

Avoidance of being bitten is the key and avoid being in areas where there is stagnant water. Professional medical care is needed in the case of infection.

See Chapter Sixteen: Prevention, malaria section

Apis and *Belladonna* may be the two main remedies initially indicated for this disease.
See Chapter Seven: Common Infections, Fever and Influenza

Lassa Fever

ONSET Symptoms begin between 6-21 days after infection. Initially looks like malaria. Later looks like Ebola.
KEY SYMPTOMS Fever, muscle aching, fatigue, slowly getting worse over one week. Extreme sore throat, lymph swelling, great prostration and pneumonia type symptoms. Blood on coughing, nose bleeding and bloody stool. Heart symptoms and meningitis and encephalitis.

This is a viral disease spread mainly through eating food contaminated with infected mouse or rats' urine and feces. It can also be caught through the respiratory tract and through broken skin in direct contact with feces. It can also spread from person to person, including through sex. There are up to 500,000 cases a year with about 5,000 deaths. The disease is more prevalent in West Africa and predominantly in rural areas. The first symptoms are like influenza, developing slowly over one week with a gradual rise in temperature, aching, headache, sore throat, etc. Symptoms then quite quickly get worse, with an extreme sore throat, glandular swelling in the throat and neck, and white patches appearing in the throat. The temperature raises more with extreme prostration and abdominal pain and symptoms resembling pneumonia. There can be blood with coughing, nose bleeding and even purple spots on the skin. In early stages it can resemble malaria and when more serious looks like ebola. If this condition is not treated quickly, there is a high percentage of fatality, so a medical diagnosis and treatment should be given. It is highly infectious so avoiding any contaminated people is important. Homeopathy can also be tried at the same time.

Lachesis is given for symptoms of an intense sore throat, prostration and any bleeding. *Crotalus horridus* can be added if bleeding is excessive. Professional care is needed.

Leishmaniasis

ONSET Symptoms may only develop up to two years after infection but symptoms can occur suddenly.
KEY SYMPTOMS Affects young children mostly. Sudden fever with periodical nature, looking like malaria. Fever continuing on and off for weeks. Swelling of liver and spleen, anemia. Skin and nails look grey. Chronic dysentery, lung symptoms, leukemia. Skin lesions, non-healing ulcers, scarring and disfiguration of face.

This is a parasitic disease spread through the bites of sand flies. There are a variety of forms of this disease, but it is commonly found in Southern Europe, Central and South America, most parts of Sub-Saharan Africa, India and China. It is frequently found in urban areas as the dog is a common vector for the condition, as can be the fox and rodents. The most serious form of the disease is called Kala azar and it can be life threatening. It predominantly affects young children and even infants. It can be very difficult to identify due to secondary disease manifestations and the fact that the incubation period may be up to two years after first infection. Therefore, if a person traveled in a foreign country two years prior and then became sick, this disease may be missed but should be considered. Often there may be no local lesion and the first symptoms will be a sudden fever with periodical highs and lows, resembling malaria. This can continue for weeks and the fever may settle to times of normalcy and then have periodic spikes of temperature. There will often be enlargement of the spleen and liver and the skin will then become very grey, especially on the face and the hands and nails. In the local population, the initial symptoms may not be as intense but will eventually develop along similar lines. One can see lung symptoms, even to tuberculosis and chronic amoebic and bacillary dysentery, as well as forms of cancer, especially leukemia. This makes diagnosis again difficult and all the more important. Inflammation of the liver can lead to jaundice and there is weight loss, anemia and swelling of parts of the body.

The fact that symptoms may appear some years after initial infection makes it challenging to diagnose. Any unusual fever, not associated with any specific infection or illness that does not go of its own accord, and if associated with weakness, anemia and possibly spleen enlargement may indicate Kala azar and needs diagnostic confirmation. However, for most travelers, it is extremely rare. Conventional treatment is effective.

● GENERAL CARE

Avoiding being bitten is crucial if in an area where the disease is known to occur. Using similar precautions to avoid mosquitoes, including the use of repellants and the use of nets, although sand flies can get through normal mosquito nets and a finer net should be used.

◆ HOMEOPATHIC CARE

The initial fever symptoms need to be treated. *Arsenicum album* and *China* are important, especially with any swelling of the spleen and liver. *Ceanothus* in a 3c potency can be given to support the spleen. Other fever remedies may be considered. Professional care is required for other symptoms.
See Chapter Seven: Common Infections, Fever and Influenza sections

⬧ HERBAL CARE

New Jersey Tea can be taken. (It is the same as the homeopathic remedy *Ceanothus*, which is excellent for swelling of the liver and spleen).
NOTE Other forms of leishmaniasis (cutaneous leishmaniasis) affect only more external areas but can still develop into destructive and disfiguring conditions. The initial bite (spread from dogs, foxes etc.) will become a hard nodule and then turn into an ulcer which does not initially heal and then as it heals over many months leaves obvious scarring. In some forms, other lesions then develop in the nose, occurring even years later and especially affecting the septum (cartilage) separating

the nostrils. The disease can then spread to the mouth, throat, larynx etc. and create destructive disfiguring of the face. The most dangerous and destructive form is called mucotaneous leishmaniasis and is more commonly found in South and Central America. It is limited to more rural areas. Symptoms lead to substantial scarring and destruction of tissue, especially affecting the septum of the nose, the mouth down to the larynx. A less destructive form of cutaneous leishmaniasis is found in Central America and also a form is found in Southern Europe, the Middle East and parts of Africa.

It is important that if any non-healing ulcer appears after being in an endemic area to get it diagnosed and treated, both conventionally and homeopathically. A professional homeopath is required in such situations and conventional treatment should be sought.

Leptospirosis

ONSET Symptoms come on 4-14 days after infection with sudden high fever.
KEY SYMPTOMS High fever, headache, chill and vomiting. Pain in stomach and abdomen, aching in body, especially the calves and great weakness. Hemorrhage of lungs, kidney and liver problems, including jaundice.

This is a bacterial disease that spreads through contact with water, food or soil that is contaminated with rats' (many other animals can also carry the disease) urine and may be found more during monsoon and flood times. It is therefore found more seasonally and in damp areas, where residual water remains. It is endemic to South East Asia and also parts of Cuba. Symptoms come on four to fourteen days after initial infection and begin with a sudden, high fever, headache, chill, vomiting with pain in the stomach and abdomen. There may be muscular aching, especially in the calf area and severe depletion and weakness. It is not easy to diagnose and may need medical attention. It can be treated conventionally and there can be serious complications, such as lung hemorrhage and kidney and liver problems, including failure. If a high fever commences with other symptoms above and then jaundice is seen, this disease should be considered. After the initial phase of symptoms, there can be lull in any symptoms and then more serious secondary symptoms are seen. It can be compared with dengue fever, malaria and typhoid.

◆ HOMEOPATHIC CARE

Arsenicum album and *Belladonna* are two remedies to consider in the initial phase of symptoms, but any of the remedies indicated for acute malaria, dengue fever and typhoid may be useful.
See Chapter Seven: Common Infections, Fever and Influenza and Chapter Thirteen: Common Tropical Diseases

Plague

The very name of the Plague illicits fear because of the history of various plagues over the centuries. However, most travelers are highly unlikely to get the plague but occasionally human cases do occur. It is spread from flea bites which are carried mainly by rats and also other rodents. If one finds oneself in an area where plague has occurred, avoid being around any rodent type animal, especially dead ones! It can also be spread easily from an infected human to another. Symptoms include a classic fever, with chills, muscle aches and a swollen and very painful lymph node, especially one that is found in the groin. Conventional treatment is to take doxycycline and there is a vaccine for those at high risk, e.g., Naturalists may consider being immunized. Avoidance of being bitten is essential through the use of clothing, flea repellent and other general prevention.

If symptoms do develop, get medical attention as soon as possible.

◆ HOMEOPATHIC CARE

See Chapter Seven: Common Infections, Fever and Influenza sections

Poliomyelitis

ONSET Incubation is up to 3 weeks from infection.
KEY SYMPTOMS Influenza type symptoms. Fever, aching, chill, sore throat. Gradually developing paralysis, including speech.

This is a viral disease well-known throughout the world for its paralytic affects, although only about 1% of polio infections end up in paralysis. Wide spread immunization throughout the world has had an impact in preventing this disease but it can still occur, mainly in developing countries. The only cases in the developed world have been through the use of live virus immunizations and people catching it from those being immunized, and also from people returning from foreign countries. A new injectible vaccine is now mainly used. The main areas where it is found are Africa, India, South East Asia and the Middle East.

The incubation period for polio is up to three weeks after infection. The first symptoms are a general lack of well-being, sore throat, aching and stiffness of muscles, especially in the back and neck. Most cases never get any worse and there is a general recovery. It may seem like a case of the 'flu. However, as mentioned, in 1% of cases, there may be a gradually developing paralysis, affecting the respiratory muscles, including speech and ability to swallow and then affecting the extremities.

Even though there have been no new outbreaks of polio in western Europe or the USA for around 40 years, some people who were exposed can develop post-polio syndrome, where they experience chronic 'flu-like symptoms and impaired neurological function. This needs to be treated by a professional homeopath or other health professional.

● HOMEOPATHIC CARE

Gelsemium is the most specific remedy for the initial symptoms of polio that resemble the 'flu.
See Chapter Seven: Common Infections, Fever and Influenza sections

Rabies

ONSET Symptoms develop mostly between 2-12 weeks after infection, but it can be as long as 2 years. However, symptoms develop suddenly and violently. Death can occur within 10 days.
KEY SYMPTOMS Fever, malaise, headache to begin with but suddenly developing intense pains, spasms in the body, especially throat, mania, rage, violent impulses, an extreme fear of water, glistening objects, convulsions and insanity.

This is a viral disease caught from the saliva of infected animals, e.g., dogs, bats, foxes, skunks, raccoons, etc. It is transmitted mainly through a bite but any break in the skin with infected saliva can be enough. Any bite from a dog that you do not know or from bats should be immediately referred to a doctor. Conventional treatment is effective if done soon enough. A rabies vaccine is available and highly effective but is not necessary for most travelers. This should be considered only for those people who could be exposed to the bites of infected animals. Precaution is important in terms of touching any dog that you do not know. It is best to avoid touching any dogs when traveling. Any wound or bite needs to be cleaned well.

See Chapter Four, Accidents, Injuries and Trauma, Bites and Wounds section

It is difficult to know if a bite from an animal could be infected. The bite may be small or even just infected saliva that is in contact with a small wound. Incubation can be from two weeks up to six months but when symptoms do appear, they can come on suddenly and violently. In some cases, symptoms may not come on for up to two years, but mostly it will occur between two and twelve weeks.

Symptoms of rabies includes a pathological fear of water (hydrophobia), extreme sensitivity to bright reflected lights and the sound of running water, profuse stringy salivation with spitting and gagging, and mental mania with loquacity, anger, rage and violent impulses. There can be convulsions and if not treated quickly, the person will likely die. However, the first symptoms are usually a general malaise, fever and headache but which then quickly develops into more intense pains, mania, spasms, convulsions and hydrophobia. Once symptoms come on, most people die within ten days.

● HOMEOPATHIC CARE

Any animal bite should be treated immediately with *Ledum*, taking one tablet three times a day for three days, alternating with *Hypericum* for three days. (This means six tablets a day for three days.) Also the homeopathic nosode *Lyssin* (Hydrophobinum), 200c, three times a day for one week should be used as prevention after a bite with any wild animal that could carry rabies. Any fever or behavioral change, including unusual fears, aggressive tendencies etc., after any bite from an animal, even months before, should be referred to a doctor. The remedies *Belladonna* and *Stramonium* can be given for any fever symptoms in which mania and rage are seen. A medical diagnosis should be done and if positive, conventional rabies treatment should be taken.

See Chapter Sixteen: Prevention, Rabies section

Rift Valley Fever

This is a viral disease spread by mosquitoes and found in South and Eastern Africa. It is usually self-limiting with the symptoms of fever, headache and muscle aching etc. The incubation period is normally within one week.

● HOMEOPATHIC CARE

See Chapter Seven: Common Infections, Fever and Influenza

River Blindness (Onchocerciasis)

This is a parasitic disease transmitted through the bite of a black fly. It is endemic in Sub-Saharan Africa and also found in pockets of Central and South America. Only trachoma accounts for more infectious causes of blindness. Millions of people are affected by this disease. Initial symptoms can involve swelling of the face with redness and itching. It is not a high risk for travelers and can be treated effectively if done so early enough. In the developing world, a lack of medical care is the main reason it is so common.

◆ HOMEOPATHIC CARE

See Trachoma Section and Chapter Nine: ENT, Eye Conditions

Trachoma

This is a form of chronic conjunctivitis found in poorer countries. It is not commonly seen in travelers but is a common enough affliction throughout the world, especially in areas of poor hygiene and nutrition. The first symptoms are similar to acute conjunctivitis. It then develops to create lumps on the upper eyelids and then the cornea becomes affected, turning grey and over a number of years scarring occurs which can lead to blindness. It can be treated conventionally, especially in early stages of the disease.

◆ HOMEOPATHIC CARE

Graphites is one remedy to consider and should be given daily for two weeks. Professional care is recommended.
See Chapter Nine: ENT, Eye Conditions

West Nile Virus

ONSET Symptoms develop 1-14 days after infection. In most cases it is a mild disease.
KEY SYMPTOMS Flu type symptoms, with fever, aching, diarrhea, headache, sore throat, lymph swelling. Occasionally becomes very serious with inflammation of the brain – encephalitis.

This is a viral disease spread through mosquitoes and which affects animals and birds as well as humans. Birds in particular have been seen to be carriers of the disease and it is found in all parts of the world, including the United States and Europe. Symptoms are similar to any 'flu, including a mild rash. In a small minority of cases, it can develop into a form of encephalitis or meningitis, which involves infection into the brain area, with much more serious consequences. Elderly and immune compromised people are more susceptible. Professional medical attention is needed in serious cases.

🌢 HOMEOPATHIC CARE

See Chapter Seven: Common Infections, Fever and Influenza sections

Yellow Fever

ONSET Incubation is between 3-6 days from being bitten. Looks similar to dengue fever and typhoid.

KEY SYMPTOMS Fever, aching, headache, loss of appetite, jaundice. Most recover after 3-4 days. A small number will develop more serious symptoms within days, including bleeding from the gums and blood in vomit and black stools leading to heart, liver and kidney failure and convulsions.

This is a disease caused by a virus, which is transmitted via mosquitoes. It is endemic in Africa and parts of South and Central America and in Africa, it is compulsory to have a yellow fever vaccine and to carry proof when traveling. It is therefore very unlikely you will see this disease but the following information is given anyway.

The disease can manifest in a mild or severe form, and the first signs are often fever, chills, muscle and bone pains, headache, vomiting and abdominal pains. Similar to dengue fever and typhoid, the pulse can often be slower than normal with and without fever. In some cases, there is an improvement after three to four days, with a general tendency to recovery. However, in other cases, the remission doesn't last and there is another rise in temperature and symptoms of jaundice appear. Nausea and vomiting can occur with a tendency to bleed from the gums and nose and black, tarry stools are seen. There may be dark blood with the vomit. There is then a fairly rapid decline, leading to coma and death. In severe cases, death occurs about 50% of the time.

Any incidence of jaundice with fever, in a person who is not immunized should be treated as a possible case of yellow fever but it needs to be compared with other types of jaundice, including hepatitis as well as malaria.

● HOMEOPATHIC CARE

Arsenicum album is one of the main remedies to consider in the first stage of the disease. *Nux vomica* is also good in the first stage when intense nausea, retching and vomiting are experienced. If jaundice is being seen, then *China* and *Lachesis* are useful. *China* will have swelling of the abdomen and great exhaustion. *Lachesis* will often have some bleeding and bruising of the skin, looking a purple color. If there is extreme weakness, prostration and great coldness, with parts of the body looking blue, then *Carbo veg* should be used. All these remedies can be repeated two to three times a day for one week or more.

See Chapter Seven: Common Infections, Fever and Influenza and Chapter Thirteen: Dengue Fever, Malaria and Typhoid

COMBINATION STRATEGY   If no one remedy is clear combine *Arsenicum album* and *Nux vomica* for the first stage of the disease. In the second stage, with jaundice, combine *Carbo veg, China* and *Lachesis*. The remedy should be given in water, one tablet of each in four ounces of water and one teaspoon taken four times a day.

Chapter Fifteen
Tick Bite Diseases

Lyme Disease

ONSET Symptoms are normally seen within 30 days of infection.
KEY SYMPTOMS In about 20-30% of cases, there is a red circular rash around bite area. This can be followed with acute aching, joint pains, fever and exhaustion. Secondary symptoms include chronic fatigue, fibromyalgia, weakness, mental confusion and weakness, Bell's Palsy and other neurological issues. Tertiary symptoms include paralysis, multiple sclerosis, mental weakness and imbalance, including psychotic states and heart pathology.

Lyme disease is put first in this section as it is by far the most significant of all tick bite diseases and needs special attention.

Lyme disease is spread through ticks by the Borrelia burgdorferi bacteria. (There are other forms of Borrelia infections from ticks and louse including relapsing fever and typhus). It is prevalent in North America and Europe but can be found worldwide. It was so-named after outbreaks of acute arthritic conditions traced to the tick were found in Old Lyme, Connecticut, USA in the 1970's. Ticks are mostly caught when walking in rural and wooded areas. Ticks have always been carriers of disease but this apparently new strain of Lyme disease has become both an acute and chronic epidemic in recent years. Acute cases are diagnosed through conventional blood tests and treated with antibiotics. However, blood tests will mostly be negative if done before three weeks and after eight weeks from the initial infection. However, if a circular rash forms around a tick bite, called Erythema migrans (EM), then one can assume a bite has occurred and it is possible for it to be infected by the Borrelia bacteria. Not all bites are infectious but given the potential severity of the disease, conventional treatment with antibiotics and also alternative treatment is recommended.

There are many people who suffer chronic consequences of the initial Lyme disease infection and should be treated by a professional homeopath or other health professional. Even when antibiotics are taken for the initial infections, up to 30% of people suffer some form of chronic consequences. That is why it is also important to take homeo-pathic treatment as well.

Diagnosis of the disease is not always clear and has become a medical controversy due to differing opinions of the disease and the challenge to obtain a positive diagnosis through blood tests. Some doctors now specialize in Lyme disease, yet conventional treatment varies widely but often involves large doses of strong antibiotic therapy, sometimes for years. However, this is not recommended by many medical authorities and the evidence to support long term antibiotic therapy is questionable. There are now various support groups for Lyme disease, some suggesting that a wide range of chronic conditions can be attributable to undiag-nosed Lyme disease.

A positive diagnosis of a Borrelia infection by a tick is done by assessing an antibody reaction with either a Western Blot or Elisa test. The tests only indicate that an infection has taken place, not whether you are or will get sick. Also, a negative test does not mean that an infection has not taken place or that the symptoms you are experiencing are from another cause. It could still be Lyme disease. There are more sophisti-cated tests now (in specialized clinics) to evaluate whether an infection has taken place which can be helpful when a person is sick but nothing is being revealed. However, in the end, it doesn't really matter that much what the tests say. Treatment should be given based on the presenting symptom picture. Doctors and other health therapists who are cognizant of Lyme symptoms should be able to evaluate it based on the history of the symptom picture, although until now, many doctors and therapists have not understood the complexity of the condition and have been unable to give many sufferers an appropriate answer to the mystery of their condition. This is especially when symptoms are in a chronic phase.

From a homeopathic point of view, it can be considered that the original infection of the Borrelia bacteria may have instigated the disease but it then activates a latent susceptibility and general immune deficiency in chronic cases, irrespective of whether the Borrelia is still active or not. Also, even if the bacteria are still active, the long term use of antibiotics can lower the natural immunity of the individual and develop greater tolerance to the antibiotics. Homeopathically, the focus is on the terrain, the individual constitution, not just the precipitating cause - the bacteria. Also, there are known co-infections, (Babesia, Erhlechia, Bartonella) as well as other neurotoxins released through the initial infection that will not be covered by the antibiotics. The impact of these co-infections varies from person to person but is mixed in with the overall symptom picture. Babesia is a parasitic co-infection and Erlechia and Bartonella are bacteria. Babesia infection can look like malaria.

If Lyme disease is diagnosed soon (within a few days) after the bite occurred, then a course of anti-biotics is generally given. (This is a more prophylactic treatment as people are mostly asymptomatic at this point and won't test positive if tested). In some cases, this is enough to deal with it. However, in other cases, it does not work and may even complicate the situation. As mentioned, up to 30% of primary Lyme disease cases continue to have symptoms even after treatment, which mostly look like fibromyalgia and/or chronic fatigue syndrome. One should still take a homeopathic remedy even if conventional treatment is taken in the first stage and constitutional homeopathic care should be sought if chronic symptoms remain after any treatment taken. This is especially the case in second and third stages of the disease when conventional treatment can be particularly challenging.

The first stage of the disease is where there is a raised red rash over the area of the bite, usually within 30 days of the bite. This may be associated with 'flu-like symptoms and aching of the body and fever. It is in situations of acute fever and joint pains that antibiotics can be effective. The second stage develops with more chronic joint, muscle and bone pains, along with great tiredness and weakness. There may also be more acute neurological conditions, like Bell's palsy (one sided facial paralysis), numbness, a lack of coordination, mental fatigue and memory loss. In the third stage, more severe neurological conditions may be seen, resembling multiple sclerosis, Parkinson's disease, severe Epstein Barre, general paresis and paralysis, and also heart pathology. Mentally there may be greater confusion, mood swings, and even psychotic conditions and deep depression. These symptoms may come on years after the initial infection and can be very hard to relate back to the original tick bite. It is only in recent years that this connection has been made to Lyme disease, making diagnosis and treatment all that more difficult.

Lyme disease has similarities with syphilis, with phases of symptom development and neurological and mental symptoms. Also the infection in both cases is a spirochete bacterium, having the shape of a spiral.

● **GENERAL CARE**

It is important to check for ticks after walking in any rural, wooded area where ticks are found. The whole of New England in the USA is a major source of ticks as are major parts of Europe, especially the Rhineland part of Germany. Any tick that is found should be removed. This is not easy and often the head of the tick can be left in the skin and become infected. Therefore, if possible try and get the tick to let go by itself or if the tick does not come off, take a pair of tweezers and gently remove the whole of the tick. Pull the tick without twisting or pulling suddenly to prevent part of it remaining. If the head does remain, it should be removed by scraping it out. Wash the area well after and use *Calendula* tincture and then cream or other antiseptic lotion, like tea tree oil. It is important to treat the bite homeopathically even if there are no symptoms. At times it has been advised to put heat or a noxious substance onto the tick. The problem can be that it will encourage the tick to expel more bacteria into the body. The best way is to simply pull the tick out with tweezers.

◊ HOMEOPATHIC CARE

Ledum is the specific remedy for tick bites and should be given both to treat any immediate symptoms after a bite or just as a preventative measure. Symptoms include a 'flu-like ache of any joints, a local swelling of the area affected, with puffiness and coldness to the part and wandering muscular pains of local inflammation to one or more joints. *Kalmia* and *Rhododendron* are other homeopathic remedies to be considered if *Ledum* does not work effectively enough after one week. The remedies should be given a minimum of three times a day for a week and then once a day for one more week. *Guajacum* is indicated when the pain is felt mainly in the bones and joints. The joints are often worse from warmth and better from a cold application although they feel worse from cold and damp in general. Pain can extend from the ankles upwards and there can be a contraction feeling in the joints and muscles with a desire to stretch. It can be given if symptoms remain after *Ledum* has been given.

A homeopathic remedy made from the Borrelia bacteria can also be given after a bite to help prevent subsequent infection. It should be given in a 30c or 200c potency once a day for three days and then repeated once a week for 4 weeks. It is not likely to be so helpful on its own for the current attack, more as prevention, but it can help the other remedies work more effectively.

Professional homeopathic and other natural medicine care should be sought when symptoms remain or develop further. It is important to treat the underlying constitution to prevent further symptoms developing. This includes when people are taking long-term antibiotic therapy. The complex and hidden nature of Lyme disease requires a comprehensive approach for which homeopathy and other natural therapies are well suited.

◊ HERBAL CARE

Teasel (dipsacus) should be taken as soon as any bite has occurred, both to treat and as a preventative measure. It can be taken as a tincture, one drop in two ounces of water three times a day. If symptoms have already developed and there is much weakness and/or pain, then it may need to be taken more slowly, beginning with one drop on the first day, one drop twice on the second day, one drop thrice on the third day, then each day adding one drop in three separate doses, e.g., (2+1+1) on the fourth, (2+2+1) on the fifth, (2+2+2) on the sixth until on the ninth day it is (3+3+3) drops. This can be taken for one month and then the dose should be reduced again. The dose can always be reduced if there is a strong reaction at any time, as it is not uncommon for there to be a dying off, or detoxifying process, called a Herxheimer reaction.

Cat's claw is another well-known herbal treatment for Lyme symptoms. It has an antibacterial and antiparasitic action. It is one of the main lines of herbal treatment against Lyme disease. Artemesia annua (sweet wormwood) is used when there are symptoms of the co-infection Babesia, which is called Babesiosis. It is a parasite which occurs with Lyme disease and often with this infection you can feel feverish with great aching in the joints. Dosage will depend on the source and strength of the herbs and should be researched when purchased.

Colorado Tick Fever

This is a viral disease spread through ticks and found in the Western United States. There are symptoms of a sudden, high fever, with intense chills and muscle aching, headache, vomiting and great weakness. The fever can last for around three days, followed by a remission for up to three days and then a relapse for another three days. This may repeat three times, followed by improvement. Occasionally, complications such as encephalitis (inflammation of the brain) and meningitis (inflammation of the meninges in the brain) can occur, but most cases recover spontaneously.

◗ HOMEOPATHIC CARE

See Chapter Seven: Common Infections, Fever and Influenza

European Tick-Borne Encephalitis

This is a tick borne viral disease, the ticks being found mainly on sheep. It is found mainly in wooded and grassy areas of central Europe and

Scandinavia. It is not a common disease and only a very small percentage of ticks carry the condition. However, of those infected it is possible for the condition to develop into encephalitis and meningitis. A vaccine is available for those at risk but side effects of the vaccine are not uncommon.

See Chapter Sixteen: Prevention, Lyme disease

Conventional treatment is also available and effective. For removal of ticks, see Lyme disease.

● HOMEOPATHIC CARE

Ledum should be given routinely for any bite (punctured wound), including tick bites, even with no symptoms. Give one tablet three times daily for one week.

See Chapter Seven: Common Infections, Fever and Influenza

Relapsing Fever

This is found in many parts of the world where the rat is the common carrier for ticks to spread the disease, as opposed to the deer in Lyme disease. It is mostly found in poor, unhygienic areas. Symptoms include a fairly sudden fever, with headache and chills, nausea, vomiting and joint and muscle pains. However, after about three days the symptoms abate only to return one to two weeks later. This cycle may continue a number of times and there may be complications with swelling of the liver and spleen and lung symptoms. Diagnosis can be important and conventional therapy is effective. This disease may also occur when lice are the carrier for the infection. In both cases, they transmit forms of the Borrelia bacteria, similar to Lyme disease.

● HOMEOPATHIC CARE

See Chapter Seven: Common Infections, Fever and Influenza and Chapter Thirteen: Common Tropical Diseases, Dengue Fever, Malaria and Typhoid

Rocky Mountain Spotted Fever

This is a typhus bacteria based disease spread by ticks and found predominantly in the western United States, although it is also found in Canada and Central and South America. It is extremely serious with high mortality rate and needs immediate medical intervention. Symptoms begin after an incubation period of a few days and consist of a high fever, severe muscular pains and headache, weakness and also great restlessness. A rash then appears after at least two days of the fever, spreading from the extremities up to the trunk, becoming rough and with small spotted bruising. Further problems can then develop, including jaundice, heart and kidney failure.

● HOMEOPATHIC CARE

Given the severity of the symptoms, it can be difficult to choose a remedy and a combination strategy may well be done, but also professional medical intervention is needed.

See Chapter Seven: Common Infections, Fever and Influenza

NOTE There are other typhus diseases spread by ticks and found mainly in Africa and India. These are not so lethal and can be treated as any other condition. Other forms of typhus are spread through louse in deprived and unsanitary situations, (it used to be called jail fever) but which will not be found in the experience of most travelers. However, historically, it has killed millions of people in times of war and other times when hygiene is severely compromised.

Chapter Sixteen
Prevention

In conventional medicine, the most common form of medical prevention is through vaccinations against specific diseases. This form of immunization is generally effective but each vaccine has its own level of effectiveness and also certain risks; details of this are discussed below.

Homeopathy and other forms of natural medicine also offer specific medicines that can act as prevention against certain diseases. These can take the form of remedies that would also be used to treat the same conditions and can be taken beforehand to help limit or prevent an illness if the risk is perceived to justify it. There are also specific herbal and other natural products that support the immune system or particular organ. There are also homeopathic preparations of the various bacteria, viruses or parasites that causes diseases. These are called **nosodes**, and are highly diluted (potentized) forms of the pathogen and are the closest analogy to vaccinations. They are totally safe and do not carry any infectious element because of the degree of their dilution but they work in a similar way to a vaccine by stimulating a specific immunity to a particular disease. Although there is not yet enough scientific data on this form of prevention, there is strong empirical and experimental evidence supporting this method to protect against an illness. It may not confer total immunity but can be part of a regimen used and can help limit any disease being protected against. This method of homeopathic prevention (also termed prophylaxis) was used by the Government in Cuba to protect against the bacterial disease leptospirosis, which is a common disease in parts of Cuba during the rainy season when infected rats' urine is spread through flood waters. A Cuban Pharmaceutical company called the Finlay Institute, which had previously made conventional vaccines, including one for leptospirosis, chose to make a homeopathic prophylaxis for the disease. This was in 2007 and 2008, when extremely heavy rainfall, including hurricanes, threatened to increase the number of leptospirosis cases. The homeopathic nosode of leptospirosis was given to over 2.2 million people in three eastern regions of Cuba to attempt to address this issue as leptospirosis can be a life threatening illness and with a population of over 2.4 million in these regions, many people are normally affected. But in 2007 there was an actual decrease in cases in December in the region given the prophylaxis but an increase in other regions not given the treatment. In 2008, there was a significant decrease with clearly confirmed scientifically proven efficacy in preventing the disease. The institute is now doing research into homeopathic prophylaxis for hepatitis A and dengue, amongst other diseases. More information on this method and the results of this policy in Cuba are described in a book on homeopathic prophylaxis, listed in Chapter Eighteen: Resources and References.

Homeopathic nosodes are used as part of the daily practice of homeopaths throughout the world. There are many others used but not relevant to this book. However, each country has its own laws in regarding access to these and other homeopathic remedies. It is best to confer with a homeopathic practitioner or homeopathic pharmacist in regard to obtaining nosodes and also which ones could be useful against particular diseases. Some will be mentioned below as part of a preventative protocol but they should not necessarily take the place of conventional prevention. They can be used along with conventional prevention or if you simply do not want to take conventional prevention, you can choose to use this method instead.

If you do choose to take a homeopathic nosode as a preventative method, try and get the 200c potency. Take one tablet once daily for three days, one week before travel, and one tablet, once weekly during your travel, taking one final tablet one week after your return. This is a general methodology, but of course, there are no guarantees and all precautions should be taken.

Having a robust immune system is the best way to avoid illness or at least to avoid becoming seriously sick, so doing what one can to establish optimal health is important. Natural medicines work by stimulating the body's own immunity, so in the process of combating illness it is stimulating the capacity of the body for self-healing. Another way is to take precautions to avoid the various bacteria, viruses and parasites which may pose a threat to an unfamiliar immune system. The decision as to what type of prevention to use depends on a number of factors, including the risks involved and the confidence a person may have in looking at all the options. In terms of choosing conventional vaccines, decisions need to be made based on the destination countries, the length of time in said countries and the overall risk involved. Often it is recommended that a wide range of vaccines be taken as a general precaution, even when the risk is very low. The discussion below seeks to give a perspective on particular risks so that an individualized choice may be made. The stages listed are somewhat arbitrary but give an idea of the risk levels involved.

The three main types of travel

1. A relatively brief (1-8 weeks) trip to a relatively safe country where you stay in a comfortable hotel or similar local bed and breakfast. The risks of most of the diseases mentioned are minimal. This can even include traveling to some more upscale places in tropical countries, including Thailand, Mexico, the Caribbean and even India. Some brief diarrhea may be the worst one can experience taking normal precautions. Very little if any prevention is needed, unless a particular risk such as malaria is known.

2. A "rustic" camping holiday or adventure trip in more extreme places, or an extended trip of months to years, often backpacking, staying in local and perhaps run down places and eating more local food on the street etc. The risks of many diseases are higher due to the exposure to contaminated food and water, mosquitoes, parasites and staying in less clean hostels/hotels. More prevention is useful in

these situations and caution against diseases such as dengue fever, diarrhea, dysentery, influenza, malaria, skin conditions, typhoid, yellow fever etc. However, many long-term travelers, even those in high-risk places like India and Africa remain free of most of these diseases by taking normal precautions. But some form of diarrhea, dysentery or giardiasis is not uncommon, as are local forms of colds and perhaps dengue fever in some areas. Cholera and typhoid are uncommon for most travelers but malaria is often a big risk.

3. A journey of a short or extended time to high risk areas, particular rural parts of Africa and Asia, or living in tropical and jungle areas of the world, where many carriers for diseases exist. People working in humanitarian aid organizations or traveling with local people in very rough circumstances and for prolonged periods have a much greater risk of contracting many of the diseases mentioned, including some of the more exotic dangerous diseases like bilharzia, leishmaniasis and lassa fever. However, anyone living for any length of time in places where these diseases exist is at potential risk.

Immunizations and Natural Prevention

Conventional immunization is achieved through vaccinations, of which there are many for illnesses found when traveling. However, there is only one vaccine that is compulsory for travel and that is the yellow fever vaccine. This is required for travel in Africa and Amazonia in Brazil and will be checked at many immigration points, especially when traveling overland between countries. (However, single entry air travel into international airports in Africa may well not be checked.) Although it is not legally required to have other vaccines, in some African countries police and immigration officials may take the opportunity to check for other diseases, especially meningitis (in West Africa particularly) and also cholera. Different countries may have different policies in this regard and although not required by law you may be asked for proof of vaccination. It can be a way for some immigration and police to make money. However, these are not mandated and it is worth checking before travel what could be expected. This is especially the case in parts of Africa.

When deciding on which vaccines to have, one should consider the

following factors
- The risks of getting the disease and the severity of disease.
- The risks of side effects of the vaccine.
- The effectiveness of the vaccine.
- The other options of protection that are being taken.
- The duration of travel.

Government websites and many other resources for vaccine recommendations tend to veer on the side of caution and therefore a large number of vaccines are often recommended. While that may seem the most effective approach, a few caveats need to be discussed.

A large number of vaccines given very closely together can upset the body's immune system and make the person feel rather unwell just before travel. In many cases, the kind of travel being done is extremely low-risk for many diseases and does not always warrant the number of vaccines recommended. It is important to research the risks and if necessary to spread vaccines out before travel and also ensure that they are done early enough before travel in case of any reactions.

If the risk is low, then maybe the vaccine isn´t crucial. Taking a six-month trip in rural Africa, working and living with people in very difficult circumstances is different from a two-week trip to Goa, India or Phuket, Thailand, and staying in a 3-5 star hotel. Always equate the level of risk involved. For the vast majority of travelers in Group 1, the risk of catching a serious disease is very slight. By far the most dangerous disease is malaria if traveling in high risk areas, especially Sub-Saharan Africa, South East Asia and Amazonia in South America.

In the United States, the Center for Disease Control (CDC) gives a lot of information on vaccines for travel as well as at home, **www.cdc.gov/travel**. They classify three degrees of vaccine guidelines: routine, recommended and required. Routine guidelines involve updating normal vaccines for children and adults, which may be recommended when traveling. That would include vaccines such as Tetanus, Diphtheria and Pertussis (Tdap), Measles, Mumps and Rubella (MMR) and Polio, as well as other recommended vaccines, which includes Varicella (Chicken pox), Human papillomavirus (HPV) Female and Male, Meningococcal Disease (meningitis), Hepatitis A and B, Pneumococcal Disease, (Lung, ear, sinus infections and meningitis), Influenza and Zoster (Shingles) in over 60's.

As stated, these are only recommendations and each country has its own guidelines as to which vaccines are recommended. The United States generally recommends more vaccines than any other developed country.

One of the newer vaccines now being strongly recommended is the Human papillomavirus for both females age 11-12 and from 13-21 years. Males not previously vaccinated from ages of 22-26 are also being encouraged. However, as with all new vaccines, the short term and long term side effects have not been established, but so far there is disturbing evidence of serious side effects from this vaccine (**www.truthaboutgardasil.org** and **www.nvic.org**).

The influenza vaccine is now being recommended for all people yearly, starting as a baby, from six months old. However, this policy is only in the United States. Most of Europe does not have the same recommendations, and the rationale for yearly 'flu vaccines is questionable. See Influenza section below.

The childhood vaccine, Tetanus/Diphtheria/Whooping cough (Dtap) is recommended every ten years with a Tetanus/Diphtheria (Td) booster. The other childhood vaccines, Measles/Mumps/Rubella (MMR) and Chicken pox (Varicella) have recommended one or two doses as a booster when an adult. It has been seen that these vaccines do not give a lifelong immunity, but as everybody is different, it is difficult to predict how long immunity lasts. Therefore they recommend a booster as a precaution and this would perhaps be offered when traveling to areas where the incidence of these diseases may be greater or when a person has not had these vaccines for any reason. Those who have had these diseases as a child however will most likely have a lifelong immunity. It is now being seen that in recent attacks of whooping cough, the majority of children had been vaccinated against the disease, questioning the effectiveness and duration of the vaccine when outbreaks occur. Pregnant mothers in the UK are now being advised to get a whooping cough vaccine as it is hoped it will give some immunity to babies, once born.

However, the Measles, Mumps and Rubella (MMR) vaccine, the

Varicella vaccine and Zoster (shingles) vaccine are contraindicated in pregnancy and for those with compromised immune systems, including those HIV positive with a CD4 count less than 200. These vaccines use a live virus in their manufacture.

Hepatitis A vaccine is a relatively recent addition as a recommended vaccine for young children but it is routinely recommended for travel, especially to developing countries. Hepatitis B vaccine is given to children, beginning at birth in the United States, but this has always been very controversial and not replicated in other countries. Its effectiveness has been challenged in medical literature and many doctors question its necessity.

The meningitis vaccine given is for the Meningococcus C strain of the disease, although just now, a new vaccine for the B strain of the disease has passed its trial stage (October 2012). There are many strains of bacterial meningitis, as well as viral forms of the disease and any vaccine only covers certain strains of the disease. Meningococcus strains A, Y and W-135 are found more in the tropics and middle east and vaccines are given for these diseases if traveling to the Hajj in Saudi Arabia and a vaccine for the A and C strains are offered if traveling in parts of West and Central Africa during certain months (see meningitis below). Meningitis C predominately affects 15-20 year olds, but overall this disease is very rare and for travel there is little risk. Young children in the first year of life are given a vaccine against another form of meningitis, Haemophylis Influenza Type B (Hib). Only one strain of the bacillus, the type B, causes meningitis. Normally, it just causes cold symptoms. It is now normally given as a combination with other childhood vaccines.

The pneumococcal vaccine is routinely given to babies to prevent lung, ear, sinus and brain infections, although the vaccine only covers a few of the pneumococcal strains that are around and therefore is not likely to be that effective. It is recommended as an adult for 1-2 booster doses although both healthy children and adults have little risk of this disease.

The main travel vaccines are discussed below.

Vaccine risks and benefits (see individual diseases).

All vaccines have certain risks attached to them as well as benefits. When considering whether to get a vaccine, weigh up the following:

- Have you reacted badly to a vaccine before, e.g., bad 'flu symptoms, or any other allergic reaction?
- Are you pregnant or breastfeeding? If so, avoid vaccines if possible.
- Are you currently sick, on medication or do you suffer from immune problems?
- Do you have an allergy to eggs? If so, avoid the yellow fever vaccine.

Discuss any health issues with your doctor or healthcare practitioner before choosing which vaccines to take. Most physicians recommend being fully vaccinated when traveling but it is important to look at the risks involved especially if you have any existing health conditions. Also, it is worth getting more information from travel experts and websites about the risks of travel to certain countries (e.g., **www.cdc.gov/travel**, a United States government site). Your local doctor may not be informed about specific risks in certain areas of travel. Also, it is useful reading books that question the effectiveness and the danger of vaccines and the ever increasing number being recommended, especially for young children. These are listed in Chapter Eighteen.

The following is a description of the main diseases found when traveling, the risks of catching them and the options for vaccination and other forms of prevention. This information may need revising due to new or different vaccines being offered so it is useful to cross-reference this information with government and health websites.

Personally I tend not to have any vaccines when traveling to India and South East Asia and when in Africa only get the obligatory yellow fever vaccine. The same applies in South America. The risk of vaccine effects has generally been played down by governments and I am generally confident of avoiding most diseases. However, it is important that each person should make his or her own decision and weigh all the options. If you do choose to get vaccinated, ensure you give yourself enough time before travel and be selective. You do not have to get all vaccines recommended to you.

The Main Travel Vaccines and Prevention Methods

It is useful to cross-reference with other health sources, e.g., government sites etc, as information on vaccine options does change.

Key: tsp – teaspoon; ltr – liter; rx. – remedy; rxs. – remedies

Cholera

Risk

- Low-risk disease for all levels. A common disease that mainly afflicts people living in unhygienic situations with poor access to clean water and food and often in some form of traumatic situation, e.g., refugees from wars etc. Only those in Group 3 of travel (see above) are really at risk.
- In case of infection, immediate rehydration is very important. Either take or make up your own rehydration liquid (1 ltr of water with ½ to 1 tsp salt and 8 tsp sugar).

Vaccine

- Although still recommended for most travelers, it is not necessary and also gives only 50-60% immunity. Only those going to high-risk areas need consider the vaccine. Some side effects can occur. Pregnant and breastfeeding mothers, and those who have had a bad reaction before to this or any vaccine, should ideally avoid it.

NATURAL PREVENTION

- Homeopathic rxs. Camphor and Cuprum 30c, one tablet of each, twice daily while in a high-risk area, can be taken. One tablet of each can be dissolved into a 1oz dropper bottle and 2 drops taken twice daily.

- A homeopathic nosode made from Cholera may also be taken in 30c or 200c potency, one tablet once weekly when traveling. Only needed when in extreme circumstances.

Diphtheria

Risks

- Low-risk disease for all travelers in all 3 groups. Bacterial infection predominantly affecting throat. Easily communicable through mucus from nose or mouth of an infected person. Incubation period between 2-5 days and disease may be passed on for up to a month.

Vaccine

- Routinely offered along with tetanus and polio in countries where recommended as part of travel vaccine protection. In childhood it is given as part of the Diphtheria/ Pertussis/Tetanus (DTaP) combination and more recently along with Polio (IPV) and meningitis (Hib). Difficult to evaluate the effects of any one vaccine as they are given in combination. Historically the Pertussis vaccine (aP) has been the more controversial, with significant side effects. However, the combination vaccine of Diphtheria, Tetanus and Polio (Revaxis), offered routinely as a booster vaccine, has seen side effects of local swelling of the injected area, with redness, pain and swelling. There may be local lymph inflammation and in some cases nausea and vomiting. 'Flu like symptoms can occur and also skin eruptions. Allergic reaction and even anaphylactic shock have been seen.

Natural Prevention

- This disease is rarely seen now. Due to improved sanitation and hygiene, the disease was declining considerably before the vaccine was introduced in the 1920's. Any actual incidence of Diphtheria should be treated with antibiotics. If you do think you may be in an area where Diphtheria is still active, you could take a homeopathic nosode, Diphtherinum 200c potency with you, and take one tablet once weekly while in that area. If the risk of infection is higher, take it daily for one week.

Hepatitis A

Risks

- Medium risk disease for most travelers in groups 2 and 3 and low to medium risk in group 1. It is also possible to catch this disease at home. For brief holidays to most places where hygiene is reasonable, the risks are slight.
- Viral infection caught through contaminated food and water due to human feces. Found in every continent. Having the disease normally confers lifelong immunity.
- There is another form of Hepatitis - Hepatitis E. Also passed on through the same route, with a similar symptom picture. However, conventional prophylaxis will not work against this strain of disease. It is common in parts of the Indian subcontinent, South East Asia and North Africa.

Vaccine

- An effective vaccine is available. This gives prolonged immunity if the full course is taken and can also be used in some cases if exposure to the virus may have taken place.
- An alternative to the vaccine is to use an immunoglobulin injection, which gives some immunity for around three months. It is not as effective but has fewer side effects than the vaccine.
- The vaccine is generally reported to be safe, but as with any vaccine, there can be both local effects soon after the vaccine, from a reaction at the vaccine site and generalized skin reaction, to more systemic effects of fatigue, weakness, fever and very occasionally anaphylactic shock and convulsions.

Natural Prevention

• Paying attention to hygiene standards when traveling is essential. Do not drink polluted water. Eat in clean restaurants. Wiping plates that are still wet may help or wash them with bottled water. Routinely washing hands when traveling is important. Avoid very greasy, oily food, especially old, rancid oils. Herbal and homeopathic support remedies for the liver are good. A homeopathic nosode, Hepatitis A is available, 1 tablet once daily for 3 days one week before travel and 1 tablet once a week during travel.

• Liver support: Chelidonium tincture or up to 3x or 3c in potency can be taken during the trip. Also Carduus marianus in the same potency can be taken, 3 drops/3 tsp., of each or 1 tablet 1-2 times a day. Milk thistle is another good liver support remedy. Different countries will also have their own natural forms of medicines. For example, in India, there is an Ayurvedic medicine called Liv 52, widely available.

Hepatitis B & C

Risk

• Low-risk for all three groups. Hepatitis B and C are viral diseases spread predominantly through blood and other body fluids. Unless one has unprotected sex, blood transfusions or uses contaminated needles, e.g., taking drugs, tattoos, etc., the chances of getting this disease are very slight.

Vaccine

• There is a vaccine for Hepatitis B but not C, including a combination Hepatitis A and B vaccine (for adults). The Hepatitis B vaccine is often given to babies at birth. However, there is much controversy over this vaccine and the risks of side effects from it. Some countries stopped giving the vaccine to babies as a result. For the first ten or more years, this vaccine contained mercury, raising concern about possible harm to the development of the brain in babies. Serious auto immune problems and neurological conditions have been seen from the vaccine. Therefore, unless in a high-risk group, this vaccine is not recommended.

Natural Prevention

- Avoidance of infection is the best protection. Avoid unprotected sex, sharing needles, even having dental treatment abroad, and getting tattoos in places that are not reputable. Take liver support remedies as above, and carry your own supply of needles should you need them.

Influenza

Risks

- Low risk for all 3 groups. The risks of getting 'flu when traveling are no greater than at home. It is not uncommon to catch a local variety of virus when in another country, when a natural immunity has not yet been established. This may often be a local cold and not really a true influenza and some immunity to local viruses is achieved once you've had it.
- Every year produces a new variation of 'flu virus and natural immunity partly depends on overall health and whether your body has some specific immunity to the type of virus. There are concerns of a new virulent pandemic form of 'flu appearing. However, even the apparent pandemic of 2010/2011 (H1N1 swine 'flu) was extremely mild and the death rate very low, questioning the pandemic classification. Much fear has been spread about 'flu and exaggerated by government, media and drug companies to increase use of 'flu vaccines but so far, nothing serious has been seen. It is hard to know if that will change. Given the normal level of risk, all 'flu vaccines are not recommended.

Vaccine

- There are currently two forms of vaccine available, the usual influenza vaccine, which is newly made each year to ideally match the current strain of virus, and a vaccine for the H1N1 strain of swine 'flu. Normally the vaccine is focused on elderly people and those more vulnerable although the H1N1 'flu affected younger people more, perhaps as older people had a greater immunity to this disease from previous exposure to the virus, even many years before. There is now research into finding a vaccine that will cover all or at least most forms of 'flu variations likely to appear as opposed to focusing only on the current strain. Some forms of the current 'flu vaccine still contains thimerosal, the mercury-based preservative, which has been controversial for a long time. The efficacy of the 'flu vaccines vary from 30-90% depending on the year, the vaccine used, the population involved and other factors. Significant side effects have also been seen with various 'flu vaccines, which may affect seniors and other vulnerable people more severely. Homeopathy can effectively treat side effects of flu vaccines. See Chapter Seven, Common Infections, Influenza section.

- Flumist is a live virus vaccine and is therefore not recommended for pregnant women, people over 50 and others with existing health problems including asthma. Due to its being a live form of inoculation, it can easily produce symptoms of the 'flu in some people. In a trial in Switzerland, it produced side effects in 36% of people, including facial paralysis in 11 people. After this experiment, the vaccine was removed from the market but in the United States it was licensed in 2003. A recipient of this vaccine may shed the live virus for up to three weeks and therefore could contaminate those close to them. Confusion has arisen how this can be avoided in daily life and from potentially exposing immune compromised people to the virus.

- A vaccine does not confer the same level of immunity as the disease itself which can give general immunity to similar 'flu virus strains. However, avoiding getting the 'flu is the best strategy. The long-term effects of taking a 'flu vaccine each year are simply not known, especially those with mercury in them. Therefore, counter to what governments and health experts say – especially in the United States – all 'flu vaccines are not recommended and are not necessary for travel.

- Antiviral medications such as Tamiflu are not recommended, being shown to have minimal protection (at best reducing the duration of the 'flu by about one day if taken within the first 48 hours of illness). There is concern that the use of vaccines and antivirals may apply genetic pressure on 'flu viruses and possibly lead to a more serious strain of 'flu developing. The Center for Disease Control (CDC) recommends it for those with more serious symptoms and for those who are vulnerable. For more information on the 'flu and the various vaccines go to National Vaccine Information Center at **www.nvic.com**.

Natural Prevention

- The best prevention is being healthy. Most forms of influenza only have serious effects in those who are weak and vulnerable, which is why the vaccine used to be recommended only for the elderly and immune compromised. (However, there is concern that a new variant of 'flu would affect people much more indiscriminately as there would be no natural immunity to it.)
- If you are beginning to get sick, take the best-indicated homeopathic remedy. See Chapter Seven: Common Infections, Influenza section. If in doubt, begin with Gelsemium. Look at the symptoms and judge the remedy on the overall picture. It will often be the same remedy for anybody who has the 'flu.
- Another more generic homeopathic remedy, Ocillococcinum has been seen to effectively prevent and treat the first symptoms of some influenza. This remedy has been verified effective in double-blind clinical trials. It can be taken immediately on signs of getting 'flu, once or twice daily for up to one week. This is available in health stores, homeopathic and other pharmacies.
- Take Echinacea in tincture for general immune support and to fight the first feelings of getting 'flu. (A good quality Echinacea will make the back of your tongue feel tingly). Increase the amount of Vitamin C and Vitamin D3. It is good to take Vitamin D3 preventatively

during the winter season if you are prone to 'flu. Ginger and cinnamon can also be taken in a tea form.
- However, in the event of getting the 'flu and continuing worsening of symptoms, do seek professional advice. Pay attention to how severe the sickness may be for others around you.

Japanese Encephalitis

Risks

- Low risk disease for all travelers. Only recommended to those traveling in all parts of Asia during the rainy seasons and if staying in rural areas for one month or more.
- Most people catching this disease are asymptomatic. Less than 1% produce clinical symptoms but acute encephalitis is the most recognized expression of the disease. Other expressions may be aseptic meningitis or general fever.

Vaccine

- A vaccine is available, but which does contain thimerosal (mercury). The vaccine is effective for two years. Two doses of the vaccine are given, one month apart and the last dose should be at least one week before travel.
- Some side effects can occur, including local inflammation at vaccine site, headache, fever, nausea and vomiting, aching of muscles, itching of skin etc.

Natural Prevention

- Avoiding being bitten by mosquitoes is the most important thing to do. (See malaria section)
- If in an endemic region and you do not want to take the vaccine, you can take the nosode of Japanese B Encephalitis, in a 200c potency, taking 1 tablet daily for 3 days one week before traveling and one tablet weekly while in endemic regions.

Lyme disease and other tick bite diseases

Risks

- Low-risk disease for most travelers in all groups, but a much higher risk when walking for prolonged periods in wooded and grassy areas, particularly where deer and sheep may live which are the main carriers of the ticks that spread the disease to humans. Vigilance is necessary and examination of the whole body should take place after possible exposure, including armpits, neck and genital region. If in a high-risk area, an insect repellant should be used. A combination of the essential oils eucalyptus and citronella may be effective in deterring ticks. Conventional insect repellant can also be used.

See Chapter Fifteen: Tick bite diseases, for removal of ticks

Vaccine

- There is currently no vaccine routinely offered for Lyme disease. A vaccine was experimentally used for some years in the 1990's to early 2000's but discontinued because of reported side effects and legal action against the manufacturer. Although the Center for Disease Control (CDC) denied the vaccine's effects, the negative publicity had its impact on demand. However, in spite of the CDC's denial, any new vaccine should be treated with caution. Medical authorities have a long history of denying vaccine effect. A new vaccine is currently under research. A Lyme disease vaccine is still given to dogs however but side-effects of this vaccine are not well documented.

- There is a vaccine offered for the viral disease, European Tick-borne Encephalitis, which is a viral disease from ticks that live on sheep. These ticks are mainly found in central Europe and Scandinavia and predominantly in late spring and summer. Most people who are bitten suffer no symptoms. Around 10% may present with 'flu-like symptoms and of these, around 10% may then develop encephalitis, an inflammation of the brain. The great majority recovers but there can be fatalities in 5% of these cases. Some cases can also develop meningitis and/or have neurological problems. Those most at risk are people walking or camping in wooded and rural areas. The vaccine is recommended to be taken every three years in high-risk areas. The vaccine should be avoided if you have an allergy to eggs or antibiotics. Children under the age of three should not get the vaccine. Children should not have the vaccine if actively sick or have a history of convulsions with fevers. Side effects of the vaccines include 'flu-like symptoms, nausea, vomiting, joint pains, swollen glands and in occasional cases, encephalitis, meningitis and multiple sclerosis.

Natural Prevention

- Avoiding being bitten is the most essential factor. Insect repellant should be used, along with checking for ticks after walking. Appropriate clothing covering the legs and arms can also help. Tuck trousers into socks and wear light-colored clothing so ticks can be seen. Ticks can rest on top of grass, up to approximately 18 inches from the ground and are very sensitive to passing humans and make themselves ready to jump. Most ticks originate from deer but it has been found also that they may come from sheep, rodents and also possibly from vectors such as fleas, mosquitoes and horseflies. There are even theories that the bacteria may be passed from human to human in the form of blood transfusions, organ transplants, from mother to fetus and from sexual contact, but this has not been proven.
- After a bite and the removal of the tick, take Ledum palustre, 30c, 1 tablet 3 times a day for 7 days as a precaution. Also take the homeopathic nosode, Borrelia, 30c once daily for 3 days and repeat weekly for 4 weeks. If the bite is with a sheep tick carrying European tick-borne Encephalitis, then a remedy made from this virus may be taken preventatively, along with Ledum. (You will have to research availability of this remedy. If bitten in summer months in central Europe and Scandinavia it is possibly this type of infection)

Malaria

Risks

- High-risk disease for all groups of travel, if traveling in a malarial part of the world. It is important to research this before travel and if conventional prevention is chosen, to take the most appropriate one. Even a short holiday to an 'exotic' place can mean a risk of malaria. Conventional prevention is most useful for relatively short trips to risky areas. For those travelers in groups 2 and 3, and living in a malarial area for a considerable time, using conventional prophylaxis is more problematic. Long-term use of more than six months can create more side effects and also lessens the efficacy. Also in the event of catching malaria drug treatment can be less effective.

- As always, appropriate professional advice should be sought and organizations such as the World Health Organization and the Centers for Disease Control (USA) **wwwnc.cdc.gov/travel/yellow-book/2012/chapter-3-infectious-diseases-related-to-travel/malaria.htm**, or the Department of Health (UK) **www.nhs.uk/Conditions/Malaria/Pages/Treatment.aspx** can be consulted to assess the risk of malaria in any given country. Parts of Africa have the most virulent strain of parasite causing malaria. Parts of Asia and the Amazon region of Brazil are also high-risk areas.

- Conventional medicines do offer substantial protection, although this is changing all the time as the mosquitoes adapt quickly to each new drug. Research into the best options needs to be done before travel. Natural alternatives or adjuncts to conventional prophylaxis do not yet have the scientific data to support their effectiveness although substantial empirical evidence in the field justifies their recommendation.

- Local people in malaria endemic areas have their own natural methods of prophylaxis and treatment. It is worth asking what they do to deal with the condition. In developing countries, young malnourished children are most at risk of dying from malaria. Adults often tend to develop some immunity to the disease and while they may get bouts of malaria, it can often be mild. Individual constitutions vary and people's susceptibility to the disease is very different. For travelers going to a malarial country for the first time, the risk of catching it is greater than for local people, although issues such as malnutrition and other immune suppressive factors can lead to a higher incidence. However, some people go and live in high-risk areas and do not get the disease. There is evidence that they have even caught the disease as shown in blood work yet remain asymptomatic.

Vaccine

- There is no vaccine for malaria at this time. Conventional prophy-laxis and treatment against malaria are as follows: (Conventional treatment can vary depending on the areas of the world and types of malarial infection. Also treatments are changing as mosquitoes become immune to drug treatment).
- The most recommended treatment now is a Combined Artemesinin Treatment (CAT). It is especially effective in treating the plasmo-dium falciparum malaria that can lead to cerebral malaria and is one of the most virulent forms of the disease. CAT is generally widely available in most parts of the world, including Africa but if you are going to remote parts of Africa, it can be useful to take some with you. Local hospitals in parts of Africa can run out of malaria treat-ment, so having your own gives extra insurance. Some resistance to Artemisin-based treatments has been seen in South East Asia while in Africa it is still very effective.
- Fansidar is a combination anti-malarial that is still used to treat plasmodium falciparum malaria. It can be used instead of CAT if the latter doesn't work. Used as a preventative when other drugs don't work, but can have side effects so is not normally recommended.
- Chloroquine was the mainstay anti-malarial drug for many years but is now used much less as mosquitoes have become immune to it. Still effective for some types of malaria, especially plasmodium vivax and ovale and often given along with Primaquine. Chloroquine also has side effects, especially if a person has existing health conditions; it is not well tolerated by many who take it.

- Mefloquine (Lariam) has been one of the main drugs used to prevent and also to treat malaria, but as with other medications, its effectiveness is diminishing. Its main effectiveness is in preventing and treating plasmodium vivax. It is taken on a weekly basis so is better suited for longer trips. It needs to be taken two weeks prior to travel and for four weeks after. As it can cause pronounced psychological side-effects, from mild to severe depression and psychotic states, including hallucinations, it is unsuitable for people with certain psychiatric conditions. It should be stopped if any such symptoms appear and is contraindicated if there is a history of convulsions. It is used also to treat malaria if the infection is plasmodium vivax or if there is resistance with other drugs to the plasmodium falciparum form.
- Atovaquone and Proguanil (Malarone, Malanil) is a newer combination pill taken daily, having fewer side effects. It has to be taken only one or two days before traveling to a malaria area and for 7 days after leaving. It cannot be used by pregnant women or women breastfeeding a child under 5 kg, and also by people with severe renal impairment. Side effects are not that common but there can be symptoms of nausea, vomiting, headache, dizziness, lack of appetite and other effects, which need monitoring. It is rather expensive and so not so suitable for long trips.
- Doxycycline is an antibiotic that is often used to treat other conditions but is effective to prevent malaria and becomes effective within two days of taking it. It can also offer protection against other bacterial diseases such as Leptospirosis and Rickettsia. It needs to be taken for four weeks after travel. However, it increases sensitivity to the sun and therefore extra protection from the sun is needed. Also, an antibiotic has its own side-effects, including vaginal thrush, and may lessen the body's immunity to other infectious diseases. Pregnant women, and children under 8 years old cannot take it. It is a cheap option as an anti-malarial.
- Primaquine is used mainly to prevent against infection with plasmodium vivax, so if that is the predominant form of malaria in a place, then this can be effective. It only needs to be taken for seven

days after travel and one to two days before travel, so is suited for shorter trips. However, as stated in the Center for Disease Control (CDC) website (**www.cdc.gov/malaria/travelers/drugs.html**), this drug cannot be used in patients who have not been tested for glucose-6-phosphatase dehydrogenease (G6PD) or have that disease, or for breastfeeding women who have not been tested. This requires consultation with your doctor and should be part of your research into various malaria preventatives.

NOTE It is important to check with medical resources what the advisable drug options for malaria are in the area you are traveling to. All side effects and contraindications should be researched, especially for those with existing health concerns and for pregnant and breastfeeding women.

The risk of catching malaria in many parts of the world is a serious one and therefore all precautions should be taken. However, it is not always advisable to take these medications for a long period of time (around 6 months) as many drugs also need to be taken for 4-8 weeks after returning from a trip making the time taking the drugs rather long. Therefore taking anti-malarial medication as prevention should be done only when there is a defined risk of catching the disease and you are traveling for a relatively short period of time. Indigenous people living in malarial countries do not take anti-malarial prevention. If they get malaria, they treat it. However, for travelers and 'ex pats' a decision has to be made if preventative medicine is to be taken and if so, which one.

On return from travel to malarial areas, be aware that malaria can manifest even up to one year later. Be aware of how you feel when coming back from holiday or travel.

Episodes of stress can initiate an attack. If you catch malaria while away, get medical advice as soon as possible. Local doctors and people will know the correct medicine to take. If you have been taking Malarone as prevention, do not take the same drug for treatment. If going to remote areas, it may be advisable to take your own supply of treatment and the correct one should be researched ahead of time. Using natural health options for prevention and treatment is highly advised.

Natural Prevention

- There is much advice regarding preventative measures. Quite simply, prevent being bitten by avoiding mosquitoes, especially at dusk and dawn. Use clothing that covers most of the body, and put on mosquito repellents containing DEET to help prevention. More natural repellents that contain citronella and eucalyptus can also be used, although it doesn't last so long. Some contain pyrethrum. It is crucial to use insect repellents. A clinical trial using a combination of essential oils as insect repellent, along with repellent sprayed nets showed effectiveness in reducing malaria. The product is called Incognito. Using mosquito nets at night is essential. Mosquito coils and other forms of 'vapor' prevention can be used but it is good not to be overexposed to their fumes. It is best to use them to cleanse the room when you are not in it. Permethrin is the chemical commonly used on clothes and mosquito nets as a repellent. It is highly toxic to cats; not so much for other mammals, but still care should be taken not to be exposed to high doses of it. Using DEET on clothes can be effective to deter bites and is good to use for mosquito nets as well.
- Take enough repellent with you, both chemical and natural forms. DEET is a chemical form of prevention, it is not natural but can be important for general prevention. It comes in various forms, a spray or roll-on. Take DEET, in 30% and 50% strength, depending on the situation. You can also take up to 75% if going to particularly malaria mosquito-laden places. However, DEET of more than 50% should not be used on babies and young children and high percentage DEET should not be used too liberally on the body. Ideally use it on your clothes, especially your socks in the evening, when mosquitoes are more likely to bite. DEET can dissolve plastics so keep it away from plastic items. Use natural repellents such as Incognito or a mixture of citronella and eucalyptus on areas around the face, neck and behind the ears. One should be very careful using DEET in these areas.
- Malaria Co nosode (in a 200c potency) 1 dose a day for 3 days, one week before leaving and then 1 dose once a week for the duration of the trip. The nosode is similar to a vaccine. It is a homeopathic

preparation of the different parasites that create malaria and its goal is to stimulate the body's own immune system in preparation for malaria infection. (Although there is no categorical evidence supporting the use of this medicine, there is substantial anecdotal evidence that homeopathic prevention in this form does work. I spent 8 months living in Ghana, often in rural areas and was bitten a lot. I didn't get symptoms of malaria although at times I was sure that malaria was incubating inside me).

- Neem tincture which can be diluted to a homeopathic dilution in the ratio of 1:10 (1x) or 2x (I drop of the 1x mixture with another 10 drops of water). Neem is called Azadirachta indica and grows freely in Asia and Africa. Making a tincture is easy and it should be taken daily, at least 5 drops twice daily during your trip and for two weeks after. This should definitely be taken along with the other choices. If you have neem in powder form, ½ tsp. can be taken daily, along with water to aid in swallowing.

- Artemesia in tincture, powder, capsules or tea can be taken as directed. This comes from Artemesia annua, (sweet wormwood) which is the plant from which is synthesized the Artmesinin treatment (CAT). Buy Artemesia tea, enough for the whole trip, plus for three weeks after returning home. Enough should be taken in case of an outbreak of malaria. For example, for a one month trip, an adult needs around 100 grams of tea, at around 1.5g of tea a day plus 35g extra in case you get malaria. Alternatively, buying Artemesia in a capsule form may be easier but perhaps not as effective. Children in general need less, depending on age and bodyweight. They may also find the tea unpalatable and other forms of ingestion are needed, e.g., capsules. Artemesia in loose powder form is an effective way of taking the herb. (Check **www.anamed.net** for information on Artemesia and how it can be taken). On one trip I took a powder with a combination of Neem and Artemesia, taking a ¼ teaspoon twice daily. So if Artemesia can be found in powder form, it can be easier to take than the tea.

- A homeopathic combination of China and Natrum muriaticum in a 30c, to be taken once a day for 3 days 1 week before the trip and once a week during the time of visit. One tablet of each can be put into a 1oz dropper bottle. (The rationale of putting more than one medicine together is simply to address the complexity of the disease, which varies in different parts of the world). Some people however, simply recommend the nosode to be used as prevention. I didn't take this protocol, preferring to take the nosode only but I did take the remedy Nux vomica in a 30c when I was feeling particularly 'liverish' and irritable.

- Chelidonium, in homeopathic dose of 3x, two drops, twice daily during the trip. This is a good liver support remedy, important to help prevent and treat malaria. The malaria parasite often sits in the liver for long periods of time and so any stress on the liver aggravates the malaria.
- It is recommended to take the Malaria Co nosode and the Neem tincture and Artemesia annua as a minimum. The Chelidonium and homeopathic combination remedies may also be taken but it is not crucial.

Meningitis

Risks

- Low level risk for groups 1 and 2 and slightly higher for group 3 if working in epidemic areas and among local people.
- There are two main types of meningitis, a viral and a bacterial strain. The bacterial strain tends to be more serious but also can be treated with antibiotics. The viral strain cannot be treated with antibiotics. Meningitis is a very serious disease and if suspected, medical diagnosis and treatment should be sought. There is a variety of bacterial strains of meningitis, some more serious than others. Childhood vaccines are given for three of these strains, Haemophilus Influenza Type B (Hib), Pneumococcal meningitis (Prevnar) and Meningitis C.
- The prevalence of meningitis for travelers is a strain of meningitis bacteria, type A and C and tends to be in parts of India, Nepal, sub-Saharan Africa, (particularly Ethiopia, Sudan, Chad, Burkina Faso, Mali, Guinea, the northern parts of Nigeria, Benin, Togo, Ghana

and Guinea Bassau), and also Mecca during the Hajj. Saudi Arabia requires vaccination against Meningitis for the Hajj (using a vaccine covering types A, C, Y and W135). Travelers to Africa are offered a combined Meningitis A and C vaccine. The incidence varies considerably and depends on location and time of year. In West Africa, there are more incidences in winter months, but for most travelers, the risk is very low. Meningitis A is mostly only found in tropical countries.

- Risk to travelers is generally slight and healthy adult travelers are not very likely to get this disease. General hygiene and a good constitution will in most cases offer reasonable protection. One should be more careful when traveling with children, especially if playing with local children who may easily spread the disease. Young children are most at risk and given that this is a very serious disease, one should always be aware of any possible symptoms of meningitis, the most significant being a high fever that doesn't abate, with head pain and pain and stiffness in the neck region with contraction of the neck, making the head arch backwards. It is painful to bend the head forward. There also can be nausea and vomiting with the headache, sensitivity to light, skin rashes, seizures and in babies, constant crying.

Vaccine

- Most children are vaccinated against two or three forms of meningitis. Travelers are recommended to get the vaccine against Meningitis A and C if spending time in the areas described where the disease is endemic, especially if spending much time with local people who are likely to get the disease. However, children who had a Meningitis C vaccine within the previous six months should not get a Meningitis A and C vaccine. The vaccine is recommended in areas where the disease is more likely. However, for most travelers, the risk of this disease is low.

Natural Prevention

- General hygiene, as always is good, but given the nature of the disease, it is very hard to avoid the bacteria or virus as the bacteria exists in the nose and throats of 25% of all people, without causing harm and giving immunity for many people. However, overall well being and fitness is a good way to avoid this disease.

- In an area where the disease is more endemic one should pay attention to the beginning of colds and 'flu-type symptoms – fever, tiredness, irritability, severe headache, photophobia and especially any stiffness in the neck, and where the head seems pulled backwards from a contraction of the meninges in the neck. There can be a rash on the body, often first occurring in the small of the back above the buttocks. Immediate medical help should be sought.

- The homeopathic remedies, Apis, Belladonna and Gelsemium may be given. See Chapter Seven: Common Conditions, Fever and Influenza section. Dissolve one tablet in water and take one or two sips, every 5-10 minutes, stirring or shaking the mixture each time. The remedies may be given separately or together, depending on the clarity of the symptom picture but antibiotics should be given in any case of bacterial meningitis. A lack of care can lead to death, especially in children. As mentioned, viral meningitis cannot be treated with antibiotics; homeopathic remedies may be used as necessary. Belladonna, in a 30c potency, 1 tablet daily for 3 days just before the trip and repeated weekly, may also be taken as prevention, especially if there is any evidence of meningitis in the area of travel.

Polio

Risks

- Low-risk disease for groups 1 and 2 and slightly higher for group 3. It is a viral disease spread through contaminated food and water, or from person-to-person through infected feces. For most cases, infection is a mild, harmless infection with digestive and 'flu-like symptoms. However, about 1% of cases can progress to the classic paralytic symptoms of polio, which in the past when there were widespread epidemics of polio led to a greater number of paralytic cases. The areas of greater risk for polio are Africa, the Middle East and parts of Asia (including India and South East Asia). There are very few cases of polio in developed countries today.

Vaccine

- There have been two forms of vaccine available, an oral live vaccine and an injectable killed virus vaccine. The latter is more often used nowadays due to polio being spread to others through infected feces or saliva from the live vaccine. The original killed vaccine also caused considerable side effects and a new injectable killed vaccine is now used. Most people who were vaccinated with either the oral or injectable vaccine as a child will have immunity to the disease in most cases. However, polio vaccine is being recommended for travelers to endemic areas. The risks for most travelers are not great. A recent campaign in Africa to give millions of children live oral polio vaccine should make travelers and those working with children in Africa more aware as the live vaccine can spread the disease to others.

Natural Prevention

- Most people who are infected with the polio virus recover with no side effects. A healthy constitution is important although there is no guarantee that this will give immunity. As the first symptoms of polio are similar to 'flu, the main remedy to consider is Gelsemium, which is also a polio remedy.

See Chapter Fourteen: Other Tropical and Infectious Diseases, Poliomyelitis section, and Chapter Seven, Common Conditions, Influenza section

Rabies

Risks

- Low-risk disease in all 3 groups. The only people at a higher risk are those working with animals in which rabies is carried, e.g., veterinarians working with animals. Animals most likely to carry rabies are dogs, cats, bats, foxes, skunks and raccoons. However, it can be highly contagious. Even an infected animal licking any broken part of the skin can pass the disease. It is important to pay attention and get appropriate medical attention if you feel there is any risk. Infected wounds must be cleaned thoroughly. If bitten, capturing the offending animal may be helpful in ascertaining if it is infected. *See Chapter Four, Accidents, Bites and Wounds sections*

Vaccine

- If bitten, the vaccine and a dose of rabies immunoglobulin will be given which gives protection straightaway. However, the issue is often the length of time between the bite and the vaccine and for assurance the vaccine and immunoglobulin should be given within ten days of possible infection. If one has already been vaccinated against rabies that can give a longer period of time before a booster dose is necessary. Being previously vaccinated precludes having an injection of a rabies immunoglobulin, which is given to stimulate the immune reaction. There are a number of different vaccines used with somewhat different ingredients. It is worth asking the doctor if the latest vaccine is being used. They are not always easily available.
- Although some people may recommend the vaccine to all travelers in countries where rabies is common, e.g., India, for the vast majority of travelers it is a very low risk if one uses common sense and stays away from animals. Also, the vaccine can be expensive and can have nasty side effects, including local swelling, joint and muscle pains, fever and more serious allergic reactions. Some people can produce symptoms of rabies, e.g., spasms in muscles and in the throat at the sight or touch of water. More serious conditions such as Guillain-Barré Syndrome have been seen. Anybody with general allergic problems, immune deficiency conditions, chronic auto immune conditions or currently having 'flu, fever or cold etc. should be very careful with this vaccine. Therefore this vaccine is not recommended for most travel.

Natural Prevention

- Avoid any animal that may possibly have rabies. Mostly this will mean dogs (and cats) that roam the streets in certain countries. Do not pet these animals even if they are seemingly tame. Avoid contact with any wild animal that is a carrier, e.g., bats, skunks, raccoons etc. Any bite from any animal should be washed thoroughly with soap and water. Follow this with Calendula and or Hypericum tincture added to some water. Once this is done, use tea tree oil to the bitten area. Any animal bite should be treated immediately with Ledum, taking it three times a day for three days, alternating with Hypericum for three days. (This means 6 tablets a day for 3 days.) Also the homeopathic nosode Lyssin (Hydrophobinum) 200c, 3 times a day for one week should be used as prevention after a bite with any wild animal that could carry rabies. However, a medical diagnosis should be made and if positive conventional rabies treatment should be taken.

- In the terrible event of developing symptoms that may look like rabies, e.g., an oversensitivity to light and bright objects, especially mirrors or reflected light, oversensitivity to running water or a fear of water, gagging when swallowing water or spasms in the throat when swallowing; spitting or frothing at the mouth, then homeopathic Stramonium should be given, ideally in a 200c, the tablet repeated hourly until symptoms may be relieved. However, if true rabies symptoms have developed, it is imperative to get all medical attention, as it will mostly lead to death.

Tetanus

Risks

- Low-risk disease for all 3 groups. Caused by infection from bacilli found in the manure of cattle and horses and spreads via a deep wound, e.g., a nail injury that goes deeply into the skin. Superficial wounds will not cause tetanus as the disease develops where there is no oxygen. Therefore, the risk factors increase when people are more likely to be injured due to adventure sports or are around animal manure that can spread the disease. There are occasional cases in developed societies but it is more common in the developing world. Tetanus is a routine childhood vaccination, so all people who had this will have some protection and do not need more unless a serious wound occurs. A booster vaccine however will give more immediate protection in event of injury.

Vaccine

- The tetanus vaccine is available in conjunction with the diphtheria vaccine and inactivated polio only (dT/IPV). It is also given as part of a combination vaccine for children. The tetanus/diphtheria vaccine is given as a booster routinely in hospitals after accidents. It is an effective vaccine but there can be side effects to it. An alternative is to take a tetanus immune globulin (TIG) after any accident, which will offer some short term immunity. If you are unvaccinated and have an injury, being given the dT/IPV is not enough to produce antibodies to fight an infection.

Natural Prevention

- Effective washing of any injury and wound is imperative and in the vast majority of cases will take care of any possible infection. The wound should be washed in warm water and soap for five minutes. Try and get the wound to bleed. Calendula tincture and/or Hypericum tincture mixed with some clean water should be used to bathe the wound. Tea tree oil can also be used. Ledum should be given 4 times a day for 2 days routinely. It can be continued for another 2 to 3 days if necessary. If pain shoots from the injured part, then Hypericum should be given 4 times a day for 2 to 4 days. If necessary, alternate the Ledum and Hypericum. Once the wound is dressed, do not change but keep it moist using Calendula/Hypericum tincture or tea tree oil.

Typhoid

Risks

- A medium risk disease, especially in groups 2 and 3. It is of no risk in most advanced societies. The areas of greatest risk are most parts of Africa, Asia and somewhat in South America, especially in poor urban areas. However, with adequate precautions, most travelers can avoid this disease. It is a salmonella bacteria spread through contaminated food and water and so avoiding any possible contaminated food and water is crucial.

See Chapter Thirteen: Common Tropical Diseases, Typhoid section

Vaccine

- There are 2 to 3 forms of the vaccine used. The older form used was inactivated (not a live virus) and was given as a course, 4-6 weeks apart. However, this vaccine, although still used in some countries, is no longer recommended in the UK or USA. Also, there can be some strong side effects from the vaccine, especially if it has been given a number of times to frequent travelers. It is also not very effective. A new live virus injectable vaccine is available as a single injection, which offers up to 80% protection. Children under the age of 2 should not get the vaccine and also those who have reacted badly to a typhoid vaccine before. A live oral vaccine is also available, taken one dose daily for 3 days. Children under the age of 6 and those with a compromised immune system should avoid the vaccine. For reactions to typhoid vaccines, see homeoopathic remedies listed for typhoid.

Natural Prevention

- Typhoid can mostly be avoided with good hygiene care. Any symptoms that seem to look like typhoid should be treated effectively with homeopathy and any other natural methods. With diarrhea, always ensure appropriate rehydration methods are taken. However, typhoid is a serious disease and a confirmative diagnosis is important to assess treatment options. The nosode Typhoidinum can be used.

Yellow Fever

Risks

- Low-risk mosquito borne disease for most travelers in groups 1 and 2 and slightly greater in group 3. The disease is predominantly found in jungle and tropical areas of Africa and South America. There have been very few deaths from this disease among foreign travelers and the vaccine is very effective in preventing it.

Vaccine

- This is mandated for travel to Africa and proof of vaccination can also be checked when traveling in parts of South America. However, one will not likely be asked for proof of vaccination when entering a country by air and coming from a non-endemic place. Apart from traveling to those countries that require it, this vaccine is not necessary. If traveling to a country that requires it and if, for whatever reason, a vaccine is not an option, a letter of exemption should be obtained from a physician. Those who are allergic to eggs should avoid the vaccine. The vaccine also has significant side effects in some who take it, varying from 'flu type symptoms to inflammation of the brain and hepatitis. It should also be avoided by those who are immune suppressed, have AIDS or cancer and are on medications for these and other diseases such as steroid medications. It should not be taken if a person has 'flu and also for babies under 9 months old.

Natural Prevention

- The most obvious prophylaxis is to avoid being bitten by mosquitoes that could carry the disease. Treating any symptoms as they arise may help curtail this disease. However, given the severity of this disease, all conventional as well as alternative methods should be applied.

Chapter Seventeen
Remedy List

Not all the remedies listed are found in homeopathic remedy kits. The most important remedies are chosen for the kits and if extra remedies are needed, they can be purchased separately, either before traveling or at the time they may be needed, if available. If traveling in more remote places or where homeopathic and herbal remedies may not be found, then the most important remedies should be carried with you.

For a list of remedies available in the homeopathic kits, and to purchase kits go to **www.thenaturalmedicineguide.com**.

Homeopathic Remedies

ACONITE monkshood

CONDITIONS Accidents and Injury, Anxiety, Bites, Burns, Colds, Coughs, Dengue fever, Ear pain, Emergencies and Disasters, Fainting, Fever, Fright, German measles, Influenza, Malaria, Measles, Poisoning, Shock.

KEY SYMPTOMS Sudden, intense and extreme symptoms. Fever high, burning, dry and sweaty, with great restlessness and thirst. Great anxiety and anguish, terror. Ailments from anxiety, fright, shock.

COMPARE Belladonna, Chamomilla, Coffea, Gelsemium.

AESCULUS horse chestnut

CONDITIONS Hemorrhoids.

KEY SYMPTOMS Hemorrhoids (piles) with sharp, sticking pains in the rectum, extending up the back. Feels back could give out. Congestion and fullness in the rectal area. Internal and external piles, bleeding, worse standing and walking. Piles with constipation and a sore, full feeling in the liver.

COMPARE Aloe, Nux vomica.

AGARICUS amanita muscarius mushroom

CONDITIONS Chilblains, Frostbite.

KEY SYMPTOMS Specific remedy for frostbite, with burning, numbness and tingling.

COMPARE Lachesis.

ALLIUM CEPA onion

CONDITIONS Allergies, Colds, Conjunctivitis, Coughs.

KEY SYMPTOMS Streaming, burning eyes, nose runs profusely, with sneezing. Dry, tearing cough from larynx, with hoarseness. Pains like needles, shooting along the lines of nerves.

COMPARE Euphrasia, Sabadilla.

ALOE socotrine aloes

CONDITIONS Diarrhea.

KEY SYMPTOMS Great insecurity in the bowel, cannot pass wind without losing stool. Emotionally a feeling of insecurity, being in unfamiliar places, not having control of situation. Stools with mucus jelly and loud flatus, sputtering and/or hot, involuntary. Pain in the back.

COMPARE Arsenicum album, Podophyllum, Sulphur.

ANACARDIUM marking nut

CONDITIONS Poison oak (ivy).

KEY SYMPTOMS Great itching, with redness and vesicles (blisters).

Numbness of skin with eruptions and after scratching. Mental irritability with itching.
COMPARE Croton tiglium, Rhus tox.

ANTIMONIUM CRUDUM sulphide of antimony

CONDITIONS Impetigo.
KEY SYMPTOMS Crusty thick eruptions, both dry and moist, anywhere on the body, especially face. Mentally cross, peevish and averse to being looked at.
COMPARE Croton tiglium, Mezereum, Sulphur.

ANTIMONIUM TARTARICUM tartar emetic

CONDITIONS Bilharzia, Coughs (bronchitis, pneumonia), Influenza.
KEY SYMPTOMS Indicated for more serious infections. Cough deep, loose, suffocating. Feels as if drowning. Fluid in lungs, respiration rattling and wheezing but little mucus raised and difficult breathing with cough. Face pale and sweating. Lungs feeling paralyzed.
COMPARE Arsenicum album, Ipecac.

APIS honey bee

CONDITIONS Allergies, Bites, Cystitis (Kidney), Fever, Hives, Japanese Encephalitis.
KEY SYMPTOMS Affected area is red, swollen, puffy or hard swelling. Intense stinging, burning pains worse from warmth and better cold. Feeling of irritation, both physically and emotionally. Allergic reaction to any bite, sting. Inflammations of skin and organs with burning, stinging pains. No thirst during heat. In kidneys, pain is bursting, with fullness in bladder and burning urine.
COMPARE Arsenicum album, Cantharis, Ledum, Rhus tox, Urtica urens.

ARNICA leopard's bane

CONDITIONS Accidents and Injuries, After Birth, Altitude sickness, Appendicitis, Burns, Concussion, Emergencies and Disasters, Eye Conditions, Fractures, Hemorrhage, Injuries, Jetlag, Pain, Pregnancy and Birth, Shock, Spinal injury, Sprains, Wounds.

KEY SYMPTOMS First remedy for all injuries and shock. Bruised, soreness of injured part. Head injuries, including concussion. For states of shock, says he is fine when not. After effects of any exertion – stiffness, sore, bruised. Fever, when feeling sore and bruised and the bed feels hard.

COMPARE Aconite, Baptisia, Hypericum, Ledum, Natrum sulph, Rhus tox.

ARSENICUM ALBUM white oxide of arsenic

CONDITIONS Allergies, Asthma, Bites, Burns, Cholera, Colds, Coughs, Diarrhea, Dysentery, Emergencies and Disasters, Fever, Food poisoning, Hiccough, Indigestion, Influenza, Leishmaniasis, Malaria, Nausea, Poison oak, Poisoning, Typhoid, Ulcers, Yellow fever.

KEY SYMPTOMS Restlessness and anxiety. Anguish and fear. Great weakness. Burning pains and discharges. Diarrhea watery, profuse, offensive. All infections of stomach and abdomen. Great nausea and vomiting and profuse watery, burning diarrhea. Acute asthma with great anxiety. Fever, with restlessness, anxiety and great chill. May have internal burning. Easily exhausted. High fever, sweats, thirst for small sips.

COMPARE Aconite, Camphor, Carbo veg, China, Rhus tox, Veratrum album.

ARUM TRYPHILUM jack in the pulpit

CONDITIONS Allergies, Throat.

KEY SYMPTOMS Allergies/hayver with rawness in the mouth and throat, desire to pick and bore at nose. Acrid and excoriating discharge from the nose. Hoarse voice worse from talking.

COMPARE Allium cepa, Arsenicum album, Euphrasia, Nux vomica, Sabadilla.

BAPTISIA wild indigo

CONDITIONS Dysentery, Influenza, Malaria, Typhoid.
KEY SYMPTOMS Serious infectious conditions, great soreness,
exhaustion and depletion. Stools dark, thin, bloody, very offensive.
Distension and rumbling. Low mental state, tiredness, confusion,
falls asleep easily, even when spoken to. Face is besotted and dark
red. Ongoing 'septic' low fever.
COMPARE Arnica, Arsenicum album, Bryonia, Eupatorium perf,
Gelsemium, Muriatic acid, Pyrogen, Rhus tox.

BELLADONNA deadly nightshade

CONDITIONS Appendicitis, Bites, Boils, Breast issues, Conjuncti-
vitis, Coughs, Cystitis, Dengue fever, Diaper rash, Ear pain, Fever,
German measles, Heatstroke, Hemorrhage, Influenza, Kidney,
Malaria, Measles, Pregnancy and Birth, Rabies, Sinusitis, Teething,
Throat Conditions.
KEY SYMPTOMS Sudden and intense conditions. Pains bursting,
sharp, throbbing. High burning fevers, thirst for sips, lemonade.
Jarring aggravates. Wild mental state with fever, pupils dilated.
Delirium. Aggression in fever. Redness of affected part, great heat.
Cough hard, intense, violent.
COMPARE Aconite, Apis, Bryonia, Drosera, Glonoinum, Stramo-
nium, Sulphur.

BELLIS PERENNIS daisy

CONDITIONS Accidents, Breast issues, Spinal injury.
KEY SYMPTOMS Injuries and trauma, similar to Arnica. Sore and
bruised feeling. Chronic effects of injuries, e.g., blows, falls, any accidents. Chronic back injury from accident. After surgery to internal
organs, to help soreness and trauma. Injuries to breasts, with residual
lumps.
COMPARE Arnica.

BERBERIS barberry

CONDITIONS Colic, Cystitis, Kidney.

KEY SYMPTOMS Kidney infections. Pain in kidney with cystitis. Pains radiating outward from kidney or bladder region. Pains felt in thighs when urinating, pains changing place frequently. Bubbling in kidneys.

COMPARE Cantharis, Lycopodium, Sarsaparilla.

BORAX borate of sodium

CONDITIONS Fungal infections, Mouth ulcers, Teething, Travel sickness.

KEY SYMPTOMS Apthae (thrush) in children who are whiny, complaining, anxious and easily frightened. Fear of being put down or any downward motion. Extreme sensitivity and starting from any noise. Thrush in nipples of nursing mothers.

COMPARE Chamomilla, Mercurius, Natrum muriaticum.

BRYONIA wild hops

CONDITIONS Accidents and Injuries, Appendicitis, Breast issues, Colds, Colic, Constipation, Coughs, Dengue fever, Fever, Fractures, Influenza, Injuries, Pain, Sprains, Typhoid.

KEY SYMPTOMS All motion aggravates, desire to keep totally still. Holds chest or head when coughing. Cough hard, dry, painful. Easily irritated, wants to be left alone. Slowly developing inflammation and fever. Dryness, especially mouth and mucous membranes. Great thirst. Delirium, saying "they want to go home", although there. Achiness, motion aggravates and worse from any jar. Injury to joints and bones with excruciating pain, worse motion.

COMPARE Baptisia, Belladonna, Gelsemium, Rhus tox.

CALCAREA CARBONICA carbonate of lime

CONDITIONS Impetigo, Mouth ulcers, Teething, Worms.

KEY SYMPTOMS Children with difficulty or late teething. Sour perspiration, especially head, timid and at times fearful. Large head, chubby. Late developing walking and talking with teething issues. Aversion to milk, including mother's. Worms that won't go away. COMPARE Borax, Chamomilla, Cina, Silicea.

CALENDULA marigold

CONDITIONS Wounds.
KEY SYMPTOMS Antiseptic and healing for wounds, especially cuts, lacerations and punctured wounds. Applied locally in tincture and creams. Given internally when wounds are painful with cutting pains.
COMPARE Hypericum, Ledum, Staphysagria.

CAMPHOR camphor

CONDITIONS Cholera, Emergencies and Disasters, Shocks.
KEY SYMPTOMS First stage of cholera (diarrhea) or fever with great icy coldness of the body, yet does not want to be covered. Abdominal cramping, great anxiety and anguish. Collapse with icy coldness. Anguish, in collapsed, weak state.
COMPARE Arsenicum album, Carbo veg, Cuprum, Veratrum album.

CANTHARIS spanish fly

CONDITIONS Burns, Cystitis, Kidney.
KEY SYMPTOMS Constant, violent urge to urinate, only a few drops being passed. Burning and cutting pains with urination. Great intensity of symptoms, cannot stand pain and urging. Blood in the urine. Second and third degree burns, extreme burning, blisters and oozing of moisture. Extreme pain, feelings of anguish and frenzy.
COMPARE Apis, Belladonna, Berberis, Causticum, Sarsaparilla, Urtica urens.

CARBO VEG vegetable charcoal

CONDITIONS Coughs (pneumonia), Emergencies and Disasters, Fainting, Indigestion, Influenza, Poisoning, Shock, Ulcers, Yellow Fever.

KEY SYMPTOMS Weakness and collapsed states. Ailments from shock, exhaustion. Coldness and yet a craving for air. Wants to be fanned. Looks like death. Lacks oxygen, turning blue. Exhausted state of any disease, much weakness, breathlessness. Great distension of abdomen. Loud and rancid burping and farting, all food turns to gas. Clothing around waist aggravates. Worse from ice cream, fruit and rich food.
COMPARE Camphor, China, Veratrum album.

CAULOPHYLUM blue cohosh

CONDITIONS Pregnancy and Birth.
KEY SYMPTOMS Erratic, weak labor pains. Pains are spasmodic, flying in all directions. Helps revive progress of labor when it ceases. Rigid cervix preventing labor. Helps prevent spontaneous miscarriage if labor type pains come very early. Good for after pains after birth.
COMPARE Cimicifuga, Gelsemium, Pulsatilla.

CAUSTICUM slaked potassium

CONDITIONS Burns.
KEY SYMPTOMS After effects of more serious burns. Useful after Cantharis has been given if pains and rawness are still strong.
COMPARE Cantharis.

CEANOTHUS new jersey tea

CONDITIONS Leishmaniasis, Malaria, Yellow Fever.
KEY SYMPTOMS Swelling and pain in spleen and liver in serious tropical diseases. Used as a tonic to support organs.
COMPARE China.

CHAMOMILLA chamomille

CONDITIONS Anger, Colic, Diaper rash, Diarrhea, Ear pain, Menstrual issues, Pain, Pregnancy and Birth, Sleeplessness, Spinal injury, Teething, Toothache.
KEY SYMPTOMS Extreme reaction to very small things. Great impa-

tience, irritability and anger, nothing will satisfy. Capriciousness. Pain out of proportion to situation. Children cannot be satisfied, shriek all the time, as if in agony. Colic, teething and diarrhea of children. Stools green, like grass, slimy, with food in, smelling of bad eggs.
COMPARE Aconite, Belladonna, Borax, Cina, Nux vomica.

CHELIDONIUM greater celandine

CONDITIONS Hepatitis.
KEY SYMPTOMS A liver remedy, with pain in the liver region extending to the back and up the right shoulder blade. Increased irritability and weakness in the afternoon. Abdominal sensitivity and bloating.
COMPARE China, Lycopodium.

CHINA quinine

CONDITIONS Diarrhea, Dysentery, Hemorrhage, Hepatitis, Leishmaniasis, Malaria, Pregnancy and Birth, Typhoid, Yellow Fever.
KEY SYMPTOMS Weakness and exhaustion, after diarrhea, fever, stool and loss of fluids. First remedy for Giardiasis. Fullness in the abdomen and stomach. Very little appetite. Easily full after few mouthfuls. Fullness, hardness and pains in abdomen and liver. Swelling of liver and spleen. Much gas, no relief from passing. Hepatitis. Bloody, mucus stool, of undigested food. Diarrhea alternating with constipation. Diarrhea worse fruit and rich food. Periodical fevers, with chill, malarial fever.
COMPARE Arsenicum album, Carbo veg, Chelidonium, Natrum muriaticum, Nux vomica, Sulphur.

CHINIUM ARSENICOSCUM arsenite of quinine

CONDITIONS Fever, Malaria.
KEY SYMPTOMS Great weakness and prostration with fever, malaria. Anemia in malaria in children. Diarrhea with fever. Mixture of symptoms of China and Arsenicum album.
COMPARE Arsenicum album, China, Chinium sulphuricum.

CHINIUM SULPHURICUM sulphite of quinine

CONDITIONS Fever, Malaria.
KEY SYMPTOMS Chronic malaria with periodical fevers, chill and weakness. Ringing of the ears and dizziness, from malaria.
COMPARE Chinium arsenicosum, China, Sulphur.

CIMICIFUGA black snake-root

CONDITIONS Pregnancy and Birth.
KEY SYMPTOMS Labor pains which are erratic and move about the body, going from hip to hip or pains which suddenly cease. Emotionally anxious, weepy, 'hysterical'. Retained placenta after birth. After-birth pains unendurable. Depression after birth. Feels caught in a 'cage' or a great cloud enveloping her.
COMPARE Aconite, Caulophyllum, Chamomilla, Gelsemium, Pulsatilla.

CINA worm seed

CONDITIONS Worms.
KEY SYMPTOMS Irritable children with worms. Great itching of the anus and violent boring and picking of the nose. Very angry and capricious. Ugly and petulant. Throws things away when given. Grinding teeth at night.
COMPARE Chamomilla, Sabadilla.

COCA coca leaf

CONDITIONS Altitude sickness.
KEY SYMPTOMS Specific remedy for altitude sickness.
COMPARE Arnica, Nux vomica.

COCCULUS indian cockle

CONDITIONS Concussion, Fainting, Fright, Grief, Jet lag, Nausea, Sleeplessness, Spinal Injury, Travel sickness.
KEY SYMPTOMS Problems from lack of sleep and anxiety and worry. Weakness and exhaustion from worry. Dizziness, heaviness in body,

especially head. Travel sickness, with nausea, vomiting and great dizziness. Has to lie down, worse on sitting, rising. Ailments from grief, fright, shock and loss of sleep.
COMPARE Gelsemium, Ignatia, Tabacum.

COCCUS CACTI cochineal
CONDITIONS Coughs.
KEY SYMPTOMS Intense, retching, violent cough. Croup and whooping cough. Cough ends in retching, thick stringy mucus coming from the mouth. Red face with cough.
COMPARE Drosera, Ipecac.

COFFEA CRUDA coffee
CONDITIONS Anxiety, Sleeplessness, Toothache.
KEY SYMPTOMS Great over-excitability, nervousness, irritability and anxiety. Sleeplessness from too many thoughts, excitability. Oversensitivity to everything, to noises, smells etc. Constantly feeling on edge. Great sensitivity to pain, especially teeth, worse touch and noise, better with ice. Weeping with pain.
COMPARE Chamomilla, Colocynthis, Nux vomica, Staphysagria.

COLOCYNTHIS bitter cucumber
CONDITIONS Anger, Colic, Diarrhea, Indigestion, Menstrual issues, Pain.
KEY SYMPTOMS Violent, intense cramping, cutting and twisting pains in the abdomen, has to bend double and/or press hands into abdomen. Restlessness with the pain, twisting and turning. Ailments from anger, indignation. Suppression of emotions.
COMPARE Magnesium phosphoricum, Nux vomica, Staphysagria.

CROTON TIGLIUM croton oil seeds
CONDITIONS Impetigo, Poison oak.
KEY SYMPTOMS Thick, rough crusty eruptions. Skin feels thick and rough.
COMPARE Anacardium, Antimonium crudum, Rhus tox.

CROTALUS HORRIDUS rattlesnake venom

CONDITIONS Bites, Lassa Fever, Pregnancy and Birth, Yellow Fever.
KEY SYMPTOMS Infected bites, looking ulcerated and bleeding black blood. Any 'septic' infectious condition with fever and hemorrhage, from lungs, mouth, skin, rectum. Puerperal fever (fever during birth or miscarriage).
COMPARE Lachesis, Pyrogen, Tarentula cubensis.

CUPRUM copper

CONDITIONS Cholera, Whooping Cough.
KEY SYMPTOMS Cramping and spasms of the limbs and of the whole body. Coldness and blueness of affected parts. Violent cough, with blueness or redness of face and spasms of body.
COMPARE Camphor, Drosera, Ipecac, Veratrum album.

DROSERA sundew

CONDITIONS Coughs, Whooping cough.
KEY SYMPTOMS Cough is racking, barking, painful spasmodic, violent. First remedy in whooping cough, croup. Retching and vomiting, red or blue face with cough. Painful cough, holds chest. Cough worse lying down, laughing and talking. Hoarse voice with cough.
COMPARE Aconite, Belladonna, Bryonia, Coccus cacti, Cuprum, Hepar sulph, Ipecac, Spongia.

DULCAMARA bitter-sweet

CONDITIONS Allergies, Fungal infections, Impetigo.
KEY SYMPTOMS Hay fever symptoms in eyes and nose, worse from damp weather and change from warm to cold. Skin eruptions, worse change of weather, cold and damp.
COMPARE Allium cepa, Croton tiglium, Euphrasia, Psorinum, Sabadilla.

ECHINACEA echinacea

CONDITIONS Bites, Wounds.
KEY SYMPTOMS Wounds that are infected and gangrenous.
COMPARE Arnica, Lachesis.

EQUISETUM scouring rush

CONDITIONS Cystitis.
KEY SYMPTOMS Great fullness in the bladder not relieved by urinating.
COMPARE Cantharis, Sarsaparilla.

EUPATORIUM PERFOLIATUM boneset

CONDITIONS Dengue fever, Fever, Fractures, Influenza, Malaria.
KEY SYMPTOMS Intense aching and pain in bones as if breaking and bruised. Aching in the back. Violent shaking chill, felt worse in back, moving up and down. Nausea and bitter vomiting, of bile. Increased thirst. Intense headache. Nausea, worse smell of food.
COMPARE Arnica, Arsenicum album, Baptisia, Gelsemium, Nux vomica, Rhus tox.

EUPHRASIA eyebright

CONDITIONS Allergies, Conjunctivitis, Measles, Whooping cough.
KEY SYMPTOMS Eyes are burning, watery and red. Simple conjunctivitis. Irritation in eyes from profuse watery discharge. Yellow/green discharge from eyes. Whooping cough with profuse lachrymation and watery nasal discharge.
COMPARE Allium cepa, Drosera, Pulsatilla.

GELSEMIUM yellow jasmine

CONDITIONS Anxiety, Concussion, Dengue fever, Diarrhea, Fainting, Fever, Fright, Heatstroke, Influenza, Polio, Pregnancy and Birth, Shock, Spinal injury, Typhoid.
KEY SYMPTOMS Fever with great aching and heaviness of the body, especially in muscles and back. Drowsy, weak, dizzy, confused and

often thirst less. Fever develops slowly. Great chills, especially going up and down the back. Eyelids are heavy, and face is besotted. The head is heavy and needs support. Anticipatory anxiety, with diarrhea, trembling. Ailments from fright, grief, shock.

COMPARE Aconite, Baptisia, Bryonia, Cocculus, Eupatorium perfoliatum, Ignatia.

GLONOINUM nitro glycerine

CONDITIONS Heatstroke.

KEY SYMPTOMS Heatstroke/heat exhaustion with extreme throbbing, exploding head. Face and skin is hot and flushed and the blood rushes to the head. Violent palpitations with or without headache, pains and palpitations worse from motion and jar.

COMPARE Belladonna.

GRAPHITES graphite

CONDITIONS Impetigo, Shingles, Trachoma.

KEY SYMPTOMS Inflammatory conditions of the eye with hardening of the tissues. Skin eruptions oozing sticky, honey like moisture which then crusts over.

COMPARE Croton tiglium, Dulcamara, Euphrasia, Mezereum, Ranunculus bulbosa, Rhus tox.

GUAJACUM resin of lignum vitae

CONDITIONS Lyme disease.

KEY SYMPTOMS Arthritic symptoms, with inflammation of joints and contraction of muscles, symptoms worse warmth. Ankle pains extending upwards, sciatica and lumbago.

COMPARE Ledum, Mercurius.

HAMAMELIS witch hazel

CONDITIONS Hemorrhage, Pregnancy and Birth.

KEY SYMPTOMS Hemorrhage after injury, e.g., nosebleeds, teeth extraction, uterine hemorrhage. Piles, that bleed profusely, feels sore

and bruised. Bleeding gums after tooth extraction. Varicose veins, chilblains.
COMPARE Arnica, Pulsatilla.

HEKLA LAVA ash of Mt. Hekla

CONDITIONS Boils, Toothache.
KEY SYMPTOMS Abscesses of the mouth and jaw with hardness around the abscess and hard swelling of the jaw. Destruction of the jaw. Facial neuralgia from decayed teeth and after extraction.
COMPARE Hepar sulph, Mercurius, Silicea.

HEPAR SULPH calcium sulphide (Hahnemann)

CONDITIONS Boils, Coughs, Ear pain, Throat Conditions.
KEY SYMPTOMS Infections with stitching, sharp pains as if a needle inserted. Sensation of splinter, especially in ear, throat, chest and skin. Pains in ear shooting to throat and vice versa, worse swallowing and coughing. Worse cold, wind and better warmth. Offensive discharge from ears. Boils and abscesses have sharp, stitching pains, worse touch and cold air. Suppurating wounds, splinters. Anger and extreme touchiness. Cough dry, intense, barking and painful. Also loose, with great rattling and hoarseness.
COMPARE Aconite, Drosera, Mercurius, Nux vomica, Silicea, Spongia.

HYPERICUM St. Johns wort

CONDITIONS Accidents and Injuries, Concussion, Pain, Spinal injury, Wounds.
KEY SYMPTOMS Injuries to nerve rich areas, with sharp, intense, shooting pains. Pain unendurable. Crushed finger tips, lacerated wounds which are very painful. Head injuries, especially to occiput, spinal nerves.
COMPARE Arnica, Ledum.

IGNATIA St. Ignatius bean

CONDITIONS Fainting, Grief, Hiccough, Shock, Sleeplessness.
KEY SYMPTOMS Sudden shock, disappointment and sadness. First remedy in acute grief. Choking in the throat, difficult to swallow and difficult to breathe, often with sighing breath. Violent weeping or can't weep at all.
COMPARE Aconite, Gelsemium, Natrum mur, Nux vomica, Pulsatilla.

IPECAC ipecac

CONDITIONS Bilharzia, Bronchitis, Coughs, Emergencies and Disasters, Hemorrhage, Influenza, Malaria, Nausea, Pregnancy and Birth, Teething, Typhoid, Whooping cough.
KEY SYMPTOMS Nausea with all complaints especially with bleeding. Cough is intense, violent, incessant and racking. Loose, coarse rattle in the chest yet little mucus is raised. Face is red with the intensity of cough with gagging and retching. Whooping cough, asthma.
COMPARE Antimonium tart, Coccus cacti, Drosera, Hepar sulph.

KALI BICHROMICUM potassium bichromate

CONDITIONS Sinusitis.
KEY SYMPTOMS Acute sinusitis with great pressure, especially at the root of nose and in cheeks. Nose obstructed, difficult to blow out mucus. Discharge thick and sticky and mucus dripping into throat from the back of nose.
COMPARE Belladonna, Silicea.

KALI CARBONICUM carbonate of potassium

CONDITIONS Pregnancy and Birth.
KEY SYMPTOMS Difficult labor with pains mainly felt in the back. A 'back labor'. Back feels as if it is going to break, give up. Labor pains unendurable, extending down the legs. Feels weak and worn out.
COMPARE Caulophyllum, Gelsemium, Viburnum.

KALMIA mountain laurel

CONDITIONS Lyme disease.

KEY SYMPTOMS Intense, sharp, shooting pains in joints and muscles. Pains wandering and shooting with numbness, in coordination of movements. Pains along nerves. Arthritic symptoms along with heart symptoms.

COMPARE Guajacum, Ledum.

KREOSOTUM kreosote

CONDITIONS Menstrual issues, Pregnancy and Birth.

KEY SYMPTOMS Chronic nausea and vomiting in pregnancy with much salivation. Chronic tendency to salivate in pregnancy even without nausea. Menstrual inconsistency. Period stops midway. Vaginal discharge burning with itching, worse before or with period.

COMPARE Nux vomica, Ipecac, Lactic acid, Sepia.

LACHESIS surucucu snake poison

CONDITIONS Boils, Bites, Bronchitis, Coughs (pneumonia), Diphtheria, Frostbite, Influenza, Lassa Fever, Throat Conditions, Ulcers, Yellow fever.

KEY SYMPTOMS Infection of left side of throat, pain worse swallowing air or liquid more than food. Lump in throat, choking feeling. Dislike of clothing, pressure on throat. Cold drinks relieve and warm drinks aggravate. Serious bites and infections on skin when purple, swollen and looks infected, turning blue/black. Snake and spider bites. Serious pneumonia with hemorrhage from lungs and skin is purplish/blue.

COMPARE Apis, Crotalus horridus, Ledum, Pyrogen, Tarentula cubensis.

LACTIC ACID lactic acid

CONDITIONS Pregnancy and birth, Nausea.

KEY SYMPTOMS Intense and prolonged nausea in pregnancy with profuse salivation and reflux of water and burning, acrid eructations.

Paleness and anemia. Nausea better eating.
COMPARE Ipecac, Kreosotum, Sepia.

LEDUM marsh tea

CONDITIONS Accidents and Injuries, Bites, Eye Conditions-injuries, Injuries, Lyme disease, Sprains, Tetanus, Wounds.
KEY SYMPTOMS First remedy for most bites and stings. Punctured wounds. Tetanus prevention. Swelling, puffiness, redness of injured part. Can feel cold to the touch. Injuries to joints and muscles and eyes. Bruising and swelling around eye. Injuries to joints with swelling, better cold applications. Prevention of Lyme disease and for joint pains after tick bites.
COMPARE Apis, Arnica, Hypericum.

LYCOPODIUM club moss

CONDITIONS Colic, Bladder, Hepatitis.
KEY SYMPTOMS For bladder and kidney conditions, especially right kidney with acute colic and kidney stones. Pains extending from right kidney to bladder. Red sand in urine, great pain passing urine. Bloating of abdomen with pains, passing of gas and aversion of clothing around the waist and back. Hepatitis, liver swollen and painful, pain extending to back and right shoulder, with fullness in abdomen, appetite less or increased, but full after few mouthfuls.
COMPARE Berberis, Chelidonium, China, Sarsaparilla.

LYSSIN - HYDROPHOBINUM (lyssin-saliva of rabid dog)

CONDITIONS Rabies.
KEY SYMPTOMS For prevention of rabies after bite of any dog, infected or not. For any symptoms that seem similar to rabies.
COMPARE Belladonna, Stramonium.

MAGNESIUM PHOSPHORICUM phosphate of magnesia

CONDITIONS Colic, Menstrual issues, Pain, Teething, Toothache.
KEY SYMPTOMS Cramping, spasms in abdomen, forcing to

bend double and better from great pressure and heat. Bloating in abdomen, loosens clothing, much flatus passed.

COMPARE Coffea, Colocynthis.

MERCURIUS mercury

CONDITIONS Boils, Diphtheria, Dysentery, Ear pain, Fungal infections, Hemorrhage, Hepatitis, Mouth ulcers, Throat Conditions, Toothache, Ulcers.

KEY SYMPTOMS Offensive taste in the mouth, or metallic taste with much salivation. Easy sweating, often offensive, and a weak depleted state. Skin looks dirty. Frequent, painful urging for bloody very offensive stool with no relief after stool. Weakness after stool. Ulcerative conditions, ulcers and canker sores in the mouth. Indicated in more serious and chronic states. Fullness in the liver region. Hepatitis. Throat infections, with swollen lymph glands, pains moving from throat to ear and back again.

COMPARE China, Hepar sulph, Mercurius corrosivus, Sulphur.

MERCURIUS CORROSIVUS corrosive sublimate

CONDITIONS Dysentery.

KEY SYMPTOMS Intense painful urging for stool with much blood and pain not relieved by stool. Painful urging in bladder too. Given if Mercurius doesn't work.

COMPARE Mercurius.

MEZEREUM spurge olive

CONDITIONS Impetigo, Shingles.

KEY SYMPTOMS Intense neuralgic pains both during and after the skin eruption. Affecting one side of the face only. Violent, irritating, burning eruptions with blisters oozing a sticky moisture and thick crusts. Worse for warmth and better for cool air and applications.

COMPARE Antimonium crudum, Graphites, Ranunculus bulbosa, Rhus tox.

MURIATIC ACIDUM hydrochloric acid

CONDITIONS Typhoid.
KEY SYMPTOMS Indicated in more serious influenza and typhoid cases, with great prostration and aching of muscles. Mucous membranes of mouth are dry, bleeding, cracked, ulcerated and the face dark red. Great soreness of body causing restlessness. Muttering with loud moaning and intense burning heat with aversion to covers.
COMPARE Baptisia, Eupatorium perfoliatum, Pyrogen.

NATRUM MURIATICUM salt

CONDITIONS Cold sores, Grief, Malaria, Pregnancy and Birth.
KEY SYMPTOMS Great sadness and grief but unable to cry, stillness of emotions. Everything feels held in, suppressed. In fevers (malarial) coming exactly the same time each day or every two to seven days. Fever with great pounding, throbbing headache, as if hammers in head. Headache from sun. Cold sores from sun.
COMPARE China, Ignatia.

NATRUM SULPHURICUM glaubers salt – sulphate of soda

CONDITIONS Concussion, Spinal injury.
KEY SYMPTOMS Chronic affects of head injury. Headaches, depression and confusion. Any condition in which a head injury initiated events.
COMPARE Arnica.

NITRIC ACID nitric acid

CONDITIONS Hemorrhoids, Mouth ulcers.
KEY SYMPTOMS Painful ulcers with sharp, shooting pains and offensive odor from mouth and nose. Cutting pains and tongue is cracked and painful. Increased salivation.
COMPARE Hepar sulph, Mercurius, Silicea.

NUX VOMICA poison nut

CONDITIONS Allergies, Anger, Colds, Colic, Constipation, Cystitis (kidney), Diarrhea, Emergency and Disasters, Fever, Food poisoning, Hangover, Hemorrhoids, Hepatitis, Hiccough, Indigestion, Jetlag, Malaria, Menstrual issues, Nausea, Sleeplessness, Spinal injury, Toothache, Travel sickness, Yellow fever.

KEY SYMPTOMS Irritation, impatience and frustration with many complaints. Intense, spasmodic and stitching pains, especially digestive area. Violent nausea, retching and vomiting. Ineffectual desire to vomit or pass stool, great urging but no stool. Ailments from too much rich food, stimulants, alcohol. Hangover. Headache with great sensitivity to noise and smells. Insomnia from too much stimulants or too much worry and excitement. Violent shaking chill, must be covered.

COMPARE Arsenicum album, Coffea, Colocynthis, Hepar sulph, Rhus tox, Sulphur.

OPIUM opium

CONDITIONS Fright, Shock.

KEY SYMPTOMS Ailments from intense fright, e.g., seeing accidents, being in war situations. Fear remains, numbness of feelings, easily startled.

COMPARE Aconite, Gelsemium, Stramonium.

PHOSPHORUS phosphorus

CONDITIONS Coughs (Bronchitis, Pneumonia), Emergency and Disasters, Female Conditions, Hemorrhage, Hepatitis, Influenza, Typhoid.

KEY SYMPTOMS Intense, hacking, tickling cough with any chest infection. Great tightness in the chest with the cough. Empty, hollow feeling in chest. Hemorrhage, of lungs, bloody expectoration with cough. Bronchitis and pneumonia. Either lobe affected. Easily losing weight with sickness. Easy nosebleeds. Uterine hemorrhage with bright blood.

COMPARE Drosera, Ipecac, Spongia.

PHYTOLACCA pokeroot

CONDITIONS Breast issues, Throat Conditions.
KEY SYMPTOMS Breasts feel hard and inflamed, with nodular enlargement, even to the armpits. Ulceration/abscess of breasts, of nursing mothers. Nipples are cracked and breast milk is deficient. For inflammation of throat, with stiffness of neck, swelling of tonsils and lymph glands. Pains worse from warm drinks and better from cool.
COMPARE Bryonia, Hepar sulph, Mercurius, Silicea.

PODOPHYLLUM may apple

CONDITIONS Diarrhea, Food poisoning.
KEY SYMPTOMS Much rumbling, gurgling and bloating in the abdomen, and also cramping, which is worse before stool. Stool is explosive and forceful. Involuntary stool, even in sleep. Fullness in liver area.
COMPARE Aloe, Sulphur, Veratrum album.

PSORINUM scabies vesicle

CONDITIONS Scabies.
KEY SYMPTOMS Great itching of skin, worse heat and at night. Stubborn scabies.
COMPARE Sulphur.

PULSATILLA wind flower

CONDITIONS Breast issues, Chicken pox, Conjunctivitis, Coughs, Ear pain, German measles, Grief, Indigestion, Pregnancy and Birth, Styes.
KEY SYMPTOMS Emotional, great weepiness, sadness and clinginess. Children who need extra attention all the time. Demanding. Yellow/green discharge from the eyes, ears or nose. Ear pain worse in a warm room, and feels better in open air. Everything better in the open air. Sadness, grief, feeling all alone.
COMPARE Euphrasia, Ignatia.

PYROGEN decomposed beef

CONDITIONS Boils, Influenza, Malaria, Typhoid.
KEY SYMPTOMS Serious, 'septic' states and fever, including typhoid, where there is intense bruised, soreness, bone pains and the odor of the body and breath is foul. The bed feels too hard. The pulse is either very quick or very slow. With fever, there can excitability, loquacity or great confusion, a sense of duality and often chills are felt between the shoulder blades. Given when other remedies are not working and the person is sinking or relapsing lower into the disease.
COMPARE Baptisia, Crotalus horridus, Muriatic acid.

RADIUM BROMATUM radium bromide

CONDITIONS Burns, Emergencies and Disasters, Poisoning.
KEY SYMPTOMS Burns to the skin from radiation exposure. Great burning pains.
COMPARE Arsenicum album, Phosphorus.

RANUNCULUS BULBOSA butter cup

CONDITIONS Shingles.
KEY SYMPTOMS Sharp, shooting, stitching pains, making one cry. Eruptions especially on the chest, making it difficult to breathe and much worse from any touch.
COMPARE Mezereum, Rhus tox.

RHUS TOX poison oak (Rhus diversoloba)

CONDITIONS Accident and Injuries, Allergies, Chicken pox, Cold sores, Dengue fever, Diaper rash, Diphtheria, Impetigo, Influenza, Injuries, Mumps, Poison oak, Spinal injury, Sprains, Shingles, Typhoid.
KEY SYMPTOMS Injuries to muscles, tendons and joints. Stiffness and pain, worse on initial motion and better from continued walking, until tired. Relief from warm applications and worse from the cold. In fevers, great achiness and restlessness. Tossing and turning at night, with pain and anxiety. Great chill, has to be

covered, averse any uncovering. Any fever with great chill, aching and restlessness.

COMPARE Arsenicum album, Baptisia, Bryonia, Eupatorium perf, Gelsemium, Nux vomica.

RUTA GRAV rue

CONDITIONS Accidents and Injuries, Eye Conditions-injuries, Spinal injury,

KEY SYMPTOMS Injuries to muscles, tendons, ligaments, periosteum and bones. Symptoms very similar to Rhus tox, with sore, bruised stiffness, which is better from walking. Injuries especially to smaller joints, elbows, knees, wrists and ankles. Tennis elbow and simple eyestrain.

COMPARE Rhus tox, Symphytum.

SABADILLA cevadilla

CONDITIONS Allergies, Colds, Worms.

KEY SYMPTOMS The nose symptoms predominate with burning runny discharge and violent sneezing. Nose itches intensely and eyes water profusely. Upper palate in the mouth itches intensely. Worms in children with great itching of nose and anus and twitching of parts of the body.

COMPARE Allium cepa, Cina, Euphrasia, Silicea.

SABINA savine

CONDITIONS Pregnancy and Birth.

KEY SYMPTOMS Tendency to miscarriage, especially at third month. Pains moving from the back (sacral) area to the front pubic region or pains shooting up in vagina. Uterine bleeding with threat of miscarriage or after birth, of dark blood with many clots. Retained placenta.

COMPARE Caulophyllum, Cimicifuga, Phosphorus.

SARSAPARILLA sarsaparilla

CONDITIONS Cystitis, Kidney.

KEY SYMPTOMS Important remedy to consider in cystitis and kidney infections. Burning pain at the end of urination. Chill in the urethra spreading up to the bladder. Gas passes from the bladder. Women may need to stand to urinate.

COMPARE Cantharis.

SEPIA inky juice of cuttlefish

CONDITIONS Nausea, Poisoning, Pregnancy and Birth.

KEY SYMPTOMS Nausea with great aversion to smell, taste of food. Nausea from poisoning, in pregnancy. Miscarriage and labor issues. Great bearing down feeling in uterus better sitting. Emotionally flat and indifferent to having child.

COMPARE Arsenicum album, Lactic acid, Sabina.

SILICEA pure flint

CONDITIONS Boils, Eye Conditions-chalazion, Guinea Worm, Teething, Toothache, Worms, Wounds.

KEY SYMPTOMS For children, who have worms with itching and are losing weight with no appetite. Become more reserved and timid and avoid company due to lack of confidence. Chilly and have profuse, sour perspiration. For splintered wounds, especially when beginning to fester. Sharp, splintered pains. Helps expel splinters and other 'foreign' objects. Mothers whose milk is not tolerated by child. Breasts are hard and inflamed.

COMPARE Calcarea carbonica, Cina, Hepar sulph, Sabadilla.

SPONGIA roasted sponge

CONDITIONS Coughs.

KEY SYMPTOMS Cough with deep, barking sound, like a seal bark or sawing through wood. Cough better cold drinks. Dryness of mucous membranes. Croup and whooping cough.

COMPARE Aconite, Drosera, Hepar sulph.

STAPHYSAGRIA stavesacre

CONDITIONS Anger, Animals(bites), Cystitis, Eye Conditions-Blepharitis, Styes, Wounds.

KEY SYMPTOMS Cystitis which begins after sex – 'Honeymoon Cystitis'. Anger with suppressed emotions, indignation and humiliation. Any physical or emotional feeling of violation. Wounds, especially lacerations to vulnerable areas, e.g., genitalia.

COMPARE Colocynthis, Calendula, Cantharis, Hypericum, Sarsaparilla.

STRAMONIUM datura, thorn apple

CONDITIONS Emergencies and Disasters, Fever, Fright, Rabies, Shock.

KEY SYMPTOMS Ailments from extreme fright, violence. Terror remains after fright. For suspected rabies or intense fever, with symptoms of intense rage, wild delirium, cursing and violent behavior. Extreme violence with unusual strength and mania. Extreme fear and terror, especially of dark, dogs and being alone. Profound aversion to and fear of water, glistening objects and reflections. Aversion to drinking water, with spasms of throat. Brain inflammations (meningitis and encephalitis) with above symptoms.

COMPARE Agaricus, Belladonna, Lyssin, Opium.

SULPHUR sulphur

CONDITIONS Bronchitis, Chicken pox, Conjunctivitis, Coughs, Diarrhea, Dysentery, Ear pain, Fever, Hemorrhoids, Indigestion, Measles, Scabies, Worms.

KEY SYMPTOMS When other remedies have only partially worked, some fever or other symptoms remain and they feel simply not right, lacking energy and interest. Great burning and heat in affected area. Offensive hot diarrhea, like sulphur. Urging for stool at 5am, or on waking. Great hunger and weakness at 11am. Mentally low spirited and indifferent. Skin looks dirty.

COMPARE Arsenicum album, Mercurius, Nux vomica.

SYMPHYTUM comfrey

CONDITIONS Accidents and Injuries, Fractures, Eye Conditions-Injuries.

KEY SYMPTOMS Injuries to bones, especially facial bones. Follows Arnica and Ledum in injury to the face when cheekbone is damaged or broken. Heals bones and given after broken bone has been set.

COMPARE Arnica, Ledum, Rhus tox.

TABACUM tobacco

CONDITIONS Food poisoning, Nausea, Poisoning, Pregnancy and Birth, Travel sickness.

KEY SYMPTOMS Deathly nausea, with white pallor, cold perspiration on the face and a great sinking feeling in stomach. Great weakness and trembling. Feeling as if could die. Travel sickness.

COMPARE Arsenicum album, Cocculus, Nux vomica, Veratrum album.

TARENTULA CUBENSIS cuban spider

CONDITIONS Bites (snake), Boils, Ulcers

KEY SYMPTOMS Ulcers and wounds which become infected, even to gangrene. Bluish/purple in color, great burning and pain. Considered for ulcerative affects of the Funnel Web spider.

COMPARE Arsenicum album, Echinacea, Lachesis.

TEREBINTHINA turpentine

CONDITIONS Bilharzia, Dysentery.

KEY SYMPTOMS Specific remedy for Bilharzia if the main symptoms are bleeding from the bladder and also for great burning in the bladder, prostate and/or uterine area. Abdominal bloating, dysentery and even colitis symptoms. Great bleeding along with burning.

COMPARE China, Mercurius, Sulphur.

TEUCRIUM MARUM VERUM cat thyme

CONDITIONS Worms.
KEY SYMPTOMS Itching of anus, worse at night. Crawling and picking of the nose. Over excitable and sensitive. Difficulty to sleep.
COMPARE Cina, Sabadilla.

THLASPI BURSA PASTORIS shepherd's purse

CONDITIONS Pregnancy and Birth.
KEY SYMPTOMS Hemorrhage, from uterine fibroids, or in pregnancy with aching in back and great bruised soreness. Intense colicky pains with bleeding. Bleeding after birth or miscarriage.
COMPARE Arnica, Hamamelis, Phosphorus, Ustilago.

URTICA URENS stinging-nettle

CONDITIONS Allergies, Breast issues, Burns, Hives.
KEY SYMPTOMS For simple burns, with only a little blistering. Pains are stinging, burning. For absence of milk in the breast, swelling of breasts. Allergic reactions on skin with hives, e.g. to shellfish and stinging, burning pains, at times with pains in the joints.
COMPARE Apis, Cantharis, Rhus tox.

USTILAGO Corn-Smut

CONDITIONS Pregnancy and Birth.
KEY SYMPTOMS Bleeding from uterus after birth, passive bleeding, with clots and dark ropy blood.
COMPARE China, Hamamelis, Thlaspi bursa pastoris.

VERATRUM ALBUM White Hellebore

CONDITIONS Cholera, Diarrhea, Food poisoning, Poisoning, Shock.
KEY SYMPTOMS The second remedy, after Arsenicum album for food/water poisoning, where there is great nausea, vomiting and diarrhea, often at same time. Feeling of coldness and cold perspiration on forehead with diarrhea.
COMPARE Arsenicum album, Nux vomica, Tabacum.

VIBURNUM High Cranberry

CONDITIONS Pregnancy and Birth.

KEY SYMPTOMS False labor pains. Helps prevent miscarriage. Labor pains extending down the front of the thighs and from the back.

COMPARE Caulophyllum, Cimicifuga, Gelsemium.

Topical remedies

The following remedies can be taken topically in either a tincture or creams/lotions

ARNICA Excellent for bruising of parts and sore muscles and joints. It is however not to be used if the skin is broken.

CALENDULA The first remedy for any cuts, abrasions and lacerations. It is to be used in tincture to wash any wound and in cream to help the healing process. It acts as an antiseptic and healing agent. (It is often mixed with Hypericum (called Hypercal)).

EUPHRASIA This is used in tincture form for all sorts of eye problems, including conjunctivitis. Can be used with Hamamelis.

HAMAMELIS This is used to apply locally to piles and for injuries, similar to Arnica and in tincture in eye problems, including foreign objects in the eye.

RHUS TOX/RUTA These are both used for injuries and soreness to joints and muscles.

URTICA URENS This is used for hives on the skin and also for 1st degree burns. It can be mixed with Cantharis for more serious burns to the skin.

Herbal and Plant remedies and Essential Oils

Essential oils can be used either topically, neat or diluted; inhaled in steam or taken as a gargle. They may be taken in a compress form. Aromatherapists use essential oils for massage. They should not be taken internally. Certain oils need to be mixed in an oil base in the proportion of 20% or less as they may irritate the skin. The proportions can be much less, even as low as about 2% of the volume of base oil. These oils include eucalyptus, ginger, lemon, peppermint, pine and thyme. Lavender and tea tree oil can be given undiluted but any irritation should still be looked for. Citronella can be used directly, along with eucalyptus as an insect repellant. However, it shouldn't be used in children under the age of three and if there are any adverse reactions they should be stopped. Both citronella and eucalyptus need to be applied every 30-60 minutes for maximum effect against mosquitoes and other insects.

There are other oils which are not mentioned here and if used should be checked regarding the amounts to be used. Of the oils mentioned eucalyptus should be used in moderation due to its potential toxicity. Water-based gels can also be used to dilute essential oils. Compresses can be hot, and used for aches, pains and abscesses, or cold and used for headaches, bruises and acute sprains.

Avoid taking strong oils such as camphor and eucalyptus when taking homeopathy at the same time. The bottles should also be stored in a separate place from the homeopathic remedies.

Goldenseal should not be taken by pregnant and breast feeding women. It should not be taken for more than two weeks in one go. Those with high blood pressure or heart conditions should not use it and if on certain medications like SSRI antidepressants, it should be taken with caution and not for long periods.

Herbal medicines can be taken in tinctures or capsule form for convenience, but if possible taken in a fresh tea form which is often more effective and cheaper. This is for leaf-based herbal preparations. Harder, more woody herbs need to be decocted by breaking down and boiling until ready. Tinctures can be taken as directed on the bottle and are a good way to use herbal products when traveling.

Essential Oils

The following are a few of the most useful essential oils.

CITRONELLA OIL This has powerful insect repellant qualities and should be used along with eucalyptus to repel mosquitoes and other insects.

EUCALYPTUS OIL This has distinct antibacterial, antiviral, immune stimulant and also insect repellent qualities. It is used to help with colds, influenza, respiratory tract infections, and on the skin to prevent infections. It is a mouth wash but is not to be digested. It should be used on the skin, along with citronella as an insect repellant. It can be applied to inflamed muscles and joints. (A recent clinical trial using eucalyptus maculate citrodora – a combination of essential oils under the name Incognito has been proven to be effective in preventing bites of malarial mosquitoes and hence outbreaks of malaria). Whether a simple combination of eucalyptus and citronella is as effective is unknown but the proven ability of these oils to offer some resistance to mosquito bites is clear.

LAVENDER OIL Used as an antiseptic and anti-inflammatory, it can be used directly on the skin in burns, including sunburn, and scalds and bruises as well as for acne, eczema, dandruff and athletes foot. It can be used externally for muscle aches, pain and arthritic inflammations.

TEA TREE OIL Used against bacterial, viral and fungal infections. It can be used directly on the skin. Externally it is useful for fungal eruptions and for injuries due to its antimicrobial action. It is one of the most widely used essential oils.

Herbs and Plant remedies

Most of the following herbs are also used as homeopathic remedies. However they have specific herbal uses and so are listed separately here. Some are given their latin name and some their common name, depending mostly on how they are commonly called.

ARTEMESIA ANNUA sweet wormwood qingaosu. This has a distinct anti-parasitic action and is therefore used in the treatment of malaria and also babesia complications in Lyme disease. The extract Artemisinin is used as part of the combination therapy CAT for malaria. Evidence suggests though that the whole plant is effective both for malaria and other conditions, such as hemorrhoids, bilharzia, chronic dysentery. It can also be used prophylactically against malaria (see **www.anamed.net** for information). It can be used both in a herbal form (a tea made by pouring one liter over approximately 2-5 grams (5 grams being the maximum dose) of dried leaves (10-25 grams of fresh leaves) and one cup taken 4 times a day), or in a homeopathic form, diluted to 6c potency in the treatment of babezia and malaria.

CAT'S CLAW It has been used in the treatment of cancer and HIV. It is an immune stimulant. It works on parasites and therefore works against the Lyme co-infection, babesia. It can be taken in doses varying from 20-60 drops in hot water, one to four times a day.

CRANBERRY It is used to help with bladder infections and is taken in a juice form.

ECHINACEA purple cone – flower. This is used for the first stages of infection, whether viral or bacterial. It also helps to stimulate the immune system. It is good for blood poisoning and septic conditions.

ELDERBERRY sambucus nigra. It has effects on the respiratory system and also the kidneys. It has antiviral qualities and is effective in colds and influenza, especially when the respiratory system is involved and with much snuffling and cold symptoms. It contains high levels of Vitamin C.

EUCALYPTUS blue gum–tree. It has strong antiseptic qualities. It works on digestive disorders, catarrhal processes and influenza. It can be given in malaria and typhoid, any condition with relapsing fevers. It is useful in kidney conditions as a result of influenza.

GUAJACUM resin of lignum vitae. This was used by Native Americans in the treatment of syphilis and therefore may be useful to be taken for the joint symptoms of Lyme disease.

GOLDENROD solidago virga. This is a very useful support for bladder and kidney infections, including kidney stones. It is also a good cleanser of the lymph.

GOLDENSEAL hydrastis. This is used for many conditions, including digestive problems, diarrhea, sinus and chest conditions, fungal infections of skin, eye irritation.

(It should not be taken by pregnant or breast feeding women or people with high blood pressure or heart conditions). It is taken internally for digestive conditions, including diarrhea. It can be used as a salve, tincture or powder.

JAPANESE KNOTWOOD fallopia japonica. This is used in Lyme

disease to treat neuro-toxin effects of the condition.

MANGO mangifera indica. Mango leaves can be used in a tea form for diarrhea and ripe mangoes eaten in cases of amoebic dysentery.

MILK THISTLE OR LADY'S THISTLE silybum marianum. This is excellent to support the liver in many liver Conditions, including hepatitis. It is also an antioxidant.

NEEM margosa bark - azadirachta indica. This has a distinct action as a prevention and also treatment of malaria. It is widely used as a food and medicine and has anti bacterial and anti viral action and is an important 'heal all' in many cultures, especially in Ayurvedic Medicine in India. It is put into toothpaste/powder and the twigs are used as brushes. It has distinct action on the skin, as an ointment or oil, being used for athlete's foot and other fungal infections, including candida and ringworm, scabies and for wounds and burns.

PAPAYA pawpaw - carica papaya. This has many health benefits, and the parts used are the skin, seeds and sap from an unripe papaya. Eating papayas in the tropics is excellent for digestive health as well as necessary vitamins. The sap is used to treat worms and indigestion and the leaves (as a tea) can be used for diarrhea and malaria. Unripe sap, mixed with clean water and salt can be used on wounds and for fungal infections. Also ripe papaya and/or the skin can be placed on wounds. (The sap can be obtained by making vertical cuts into an unripe papaya while it is still on the tree. Collect the sap into a cup (about 4 tsp for an adult and 1-2 tsp for a child). Ensure the knife is clean and wash the papaya first). Mix the sap into clean water, both for topical use and for taking internally.

ST. MARY'S THISTLE carduus marianus. This is a specific remedy for the liver and spleen. It assists in any inflammation, swelling and pain in the liver, whether due to acute hepatitis or chronic problems of the liver due to alcoholism and for any spleen affection. It is given in both tincture and in homeopathic form.

TEASEL dipsacus. A common plant which is effective in the treatment of Lyme disease and other bacterial conditions.

UVA URSI bearberry. This is used in urinary conditions against bladder infections.

VALERIAN valeriana. This is good for general states of anxiety, nervousness, nerve pains and insomnia.

VERVAINE verbena officianalis. This helps lactating women produce more milk. It is also good for general exhaustion and nervousness, headaches and also upset digestion.

Chapter Eighteen
Resources And References

For information on ordering books, kits and other information go to **www.thenaturalmedicineguide.com**.

TRAVEL BOOKS

- *The World Traveller's Manual of Homeopathy* – Dr. Colin Lessell. An excellent resource with homeopathic suggestions and overview of many conditions facing travelers.
- *The Tropical Traveller, The Essential Guide to Travel in Hot Countries* – John Hatt. A hugely informative book on most of the things a person could come across when traveling. Focusing on tropical travel, it also covers many practical and also unusual circumstances in which travelers may find themselves.
- *Where There is No Doctor* – David Werner. The essential emergency medical guide for anybody out there without medical backup. For anybody working in any capacity in developing countries, this book is a wealth of information. (Available as a PDF and in book form from the Hesparian Foundation. **www.hesparian.org**)
- *How to Shit Around The World – The Art of Staying Clean and Healthy While Traveling* – Dr Jane Wilson-Howarth. The book

to prepare any traveler what to expect when faced with dealing with this essential human function in unusual circumstances.

VACCINES AND PROPHYLAXIS.

- *The Vaccine Guide, Making an informed choice* - Randall Neustaedter. One of the most comprehensive guides to all vaccines.
- *Vaccines, Are They Really Safe and Effective* - Neil Z. Miller. A concise yet thorough analysis of the effects of vaccines, with full documentation of all his sources.
- *A history of the 'flu* - Randall Neustaedter. An excellent historical summary of the 'flu and its effects.
- *A Handbook of Homeopathic Alternatives to Immunization* - Susan Curtis. A homeopathic perspective on what homeopathy offers instead of conventional immunizations.
- *The No Nonsense Travel Vaccine Handbook*, A practical Guide for Travelers - Liz Bevan-Jones and Yvonne Stone. A detailed and practical guide on vaccines and their effects for travelers.
- *The Complete Practitioner's Manual of Homeoprophylaxis* - Dr Isaac Golden. A thorough scientific analysis of the concept of homeoprophyaxis, how homeopathic remedies can prevent disease as well as cure.
- National Vaccine Information Center - **www.nvic.org** National organization in the United States that has much information on all vaccine issues.

HOMEOPATHY BOOKS

- *Everybody's Guide to Homeopathic Medicines* - Dana Ullman and Stephen Cummings. An excellent overview of homeopathy and how it can be used on a daily basis by one and all.
- *Impossible Cure, The Promise of Homeopathy* - Amy Lansky. One of the most comprehensive introductions to the history and philosophy of homeopathy.
- *The Homeopathic Treatment of Influenza, Surviving Epidemics and Pandemics, Past, Present and Future with Homeopathy*

- Sandra J. Perko, PhD. A fascinating exploration of the 1918 influenza epidemic and how homeopathy worked to treat the disease, with comments on its ability to treat similar epidemics now and in the future.
- *Your Natural Medicine Cabinet* – Burke Lennihan. An excellent introduction to homeopathy and other natural healing methods.
- *The Organon of the Healing Art* – Samuel Hahnemann – Edited by Wenda Brewster O'Reilly. The best modern interpretation of Samuel Hahnemann's (the founder of homeopathy) seminal contribution to medical thought.

The Vaccine and Homeopathy books are all available at homeopathic bookstores and pharmacies listed.

OTHER BOOKS

- *Lyme Disease, Healing Lyme Disease Naturally* - Wolf Storl.

WEBSITES

Health and international travel/vaccine websites

World Health Organization

- www.who.int/en
- www.who.int/itch/vaccines/en

USA Center for Disease Control

- www.cdc.gov
- www.cdc.gov/travel/page/vaccinations.htm

International Association for Medical Assistance to Travelers (IAMAT)

- www.iamat.org

Gives information on health risks, information on diseases throughout the world, vaccine information and lists of doctors throughout the world.

- www.fco.gov.uk/en/travel-and-living-abroad/staying-safe/health

Anamed (Action for Natural Medicine)

- www.anamed.net.

A Christian organization working primarily in Africa that facilitates the use of natural medicine to support and treat many tropical conditions, including malaria and HIV/AIDS. They especially advocate the use of Artemesia annua (the natural source of the Artemisinin based malaria treatments) and of Moringa as a food supplement for all people, including those with HIV.

Most governments of most countries will have their own website dedicated to giving information to people traveling in foreign countries.

Travel book publishers such as Moon Books, Lonely Planet, Bradt Guides and Rough Guide Books also have health information on their websites and in their books.

Homeopathic Remedies

Homeopathic remedies are freely available over the counter in many countries of the world. However, each country has its own laws regarding this. Also, in some countries, remedies such as homeopathic nosodes are only available with a prescription.

The following is a summary of the general availability of remedies.

UK Remedies are freely available and are found in specific homeopathic pharmacies, health food stores and general pharmacies. Potencies above 30c may need to be bought from a homeopathic pharmacy.

WESTERN EUROPE France has a very wide access to homeopathic remedies and are found in most pharmacies. However, one cannot find potencies above 30c. Germany also has easy access to homeopathic remedies and also has some excellent homeopathic pharmacies where remedies can be ordered from. The same applies in Holland and also in Scandinavia. In Spain and Portugal, remedies are not that available but one can order them through certain pharmacies. They can be found however in larger cities in health food stores. In Italy a limited range of homeopathic remedies may often be bought in local pharmacies in potencies up to a 30c.

NORTH AMERICA Homeopathic remedies are freely available and found in health food stores and specialized pharmacies. They are not found in general pharmacies. There are homeopathic pharmacies on both the East and West coasts of the country and most remedies can be ordered online or on the phone. Remedies will not be commonly found in smaller towns and cities or in rural areas.

CENTRAL AND SOUTH AMERICA Homeopathic remedies are commonly found throughout the continent. They can be found both in homeopathic pharmacies and other general pharmacies, depending where you are. Major cities will have much more availability. In Brazil, one should have a prescription from a homeopathic doctor to get a homeopathic remedy although by law homeopathic pharmacies can sell remedies in a 6c potency.

AUSTRALIA AND NEW ZEALAND Homeopathic remedies are freely available and found in health food stores, certain pharmacies and from specific homeopathic pharmacies or from homeopathic practitioners.

RUSSIA AND SURROUNDING REGION Homeopathy is practiced in Russia and therefore homeopathic remedies can be found, but it is not that easy and you will have to ask where you can get them. Again, major cities are going to be easier than more remote places.

AFRICA Outside South Africa, homeopathic remedies are not available in the vast majority of places. Perhaps in major cities one can find them but there are no guarantees.

INDIAN SUBCONTINENT Homeopathy is widely practiced, and therefore remedies are available easily from pharmacies and homeopathic clinics throughout India, Pakistan, Bangladesh and Sri Lanka.

Pharmacies and Supplies

USA

- Hahnemann Laboratories Inc San Rafael, California
  www.hahnemannlabs.com Tel 415-451-6978
- Homeopathic Educational Services, Berkeley, California.

www.homeopathic.com Tel 510-649-0294
- Homeopathy World
  www.homeopathyworld.com Tel Toll Free 866-346-5105
  805-633-4737
- Natural Health Supply, Santa Fe, New Mexico.
  www.a2zhomeopathy.com Tel 800-689-1608
- Washington Homeopathic Products
  www.homeopathyworks.com Tel 304-258-2541,
  800-336-1695
- Wholehealthnow.com Tel 707-822-5807, Books
  - 866-599-5950

UK

- Ainsworth's Homeopathic Pharmacy, London.
  www.ainsworths.com Tel 020-7935 -5330 01883-340332
- Helios Homeopathic Pharmacy, Tunbridge Wells, Kent.
  www.helios.co.uk Tel 01892- 537254
- The Homeopathic Book Company, Grantham.
  www.homeopathicbooks.co.uk Tel 01476-550754
- Minerva Books, Trowbridge, Wiltshire
  www.minervabooks.co.uk Tel 01225-760003

Homeopathic Organizations

USA

- National Center of Homeopathy, Washington D.C. www.
  homeopathic.org.
- Council for Homeopathic Certification. (Practitioner listings)
  www.homeopathicdirectory.com

UK

- Society of Homeopaths
  www.homeopathy-soh.org

Index Of Conditions

A.

Abdominal pain 71
Abscess - *See Boils and Toothache* 124,141
Accidents and injury 33
African Sleeping Sickness 167, 174
After Birth 133
Allergies 113
Altitude Sickness 36
American Trypanosomiasis - *See Chagas disease* 168, 178
Anger 65
Animals (bedbugs, lice, fleas) 140
Anxiety 66
Appendicitis 71

B.

Back injury - *See Spinal injury* 60
Before Birth 129
Bedbugs - *See Animals* 140
Bilharzia 168, 175
Birth - *See Pregnancy and Birth* 129
Bites 37
Bleeding - *See Hemorrhage* 51
Blepharitis 118

Boils 141
Breast issues - *including injury* 127
Bronchitis - *See Coughs* 108
Brucellosis 168, 177
Burns 43

C.

Chagas disease 168, 178
Chalazion 119
Chicken pox 101
Children's Diseases 101
Chilblains 143
Cholera 169, 179
Colorado Tick Fever 202
Colds 107
Coldsores 115
Colic 73
Collapse - *See Shock* 56
Concussion 45
Conjunctivitis 118
Constipation 74
Coughs 108
Cystitis 135

D.
Dengue Fever 153, 154
Diphtheria 169, 181
Diaper rash 75
Diarrhea 75
Dysentery 79

E.
Ear pain & Injury 118
Emergencies and Disaster 46
European Tick Borne-Encephalitis - *See Fever* 202
Eye conditions & Injury 118-120

F.
Fainting 48
Fever 93
Filiariasis 169, 181
Fleas - *See Animals* 140
Food poisoning 82
Fractures 48
Fright 67
Frostbite 49
Fungal infections 143

G.
German measles 102
Grief 68
Guinea Worm 169, 182

H.
Hangover 50
Headache 50
Heatstroke 51
Hemorrhage 52
Hemorrhoids 83
Hepatitis 84
Herpes - *See Cold sores and Female conditions* 115, 127
Hives 145
Hookworm Disease 170, 183

Human African Trypanosomiasis - *See African Sleeping Sickness* 167, 184

I.
Impetigo 146
Indigestion 87
Influenza 96
Injuries - *See Accidents and Injuries* 33
Insomnia - *See Sleeplessness* 58

J.
Japanese Encephalitis 170, 184
Jetlag 53

L.
Lassa Fever 170, 185
Leishmaniasis 170, 186
Leptospirosis 170, 188
Lice - *See Animals* 140
Lyme disease 00, 00

M.
Malaria 153, 155
Measles 102
Menstrual issues 128
Miscarriage 131
Mouth ulcers 120
Mumps 103

N.
Nausea - *See Pregnancy and Birth* 130

O.
Onchocerciasis - *See River Blindness* 172, 192

P.
Pain 54
Piles - *See Hemorrhoids* 83
Plague 171, 189
Polio 171, 190

Poisoning 55
Poison oak/ivy 147
Pneumonia - *See Coughs* 108
Pregnancy and Birth 129

R.

Rabies 172, 191
Relapsing Fever 203
Rift Valley Fever 172, 192
River Blindness 172, 192
Rocky Mountain Spotted Fever 204

S.

Scabies 148
Shistosomiasis - *See Bilharzia* 168, 175
Shingles 149
Shock 56
Sinusitis 121
Sleeplessness 58
Snake bites - *See Bites* 37
Spinal Injury 60
Sprains 60
Strains - *See Accidents, Sprains* 60
Styes 119
Sunburn - *See Burns and Heatstroke* 45
Sunstroke - *See Heatstroke* 52
Surgery 61

T.

Teething 122
Tick bites - *See Bites, Lyme disease* 37, 197
Throat conditions 123
Toothache 124
Trachoma 174, 193
Travel Sickness 62
Typhoid 154, 162

U.

Ulcers 150

V.

Vaginal conditions - *See Women's conditions* 127

W.

West Nile Virus 173, 193
Whooping cough 104l, 108
Women's conditions 127
Worms 89
Wounds 62

Y.

Yellow Fever 173, 194

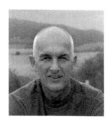

Richard Pitt has practiced homeopathy for over 30 years. He originally trained and practiced in the U.K. and then moved to the United States. He also studied homeopathy in Greece and India. He has been involved with homeopathic education for many years, running a school in San Francisco for 12 years, and also teaching throughout the country. He was involved with the development of standards of practice and education, serving on the board of the Council for Homeopathic Certification for 17 years, which has established the largest accreditation organization in North America. He also served on the boards of the Council for Homeopathic Education and the California Health Freedom Coalition, which established the legal framework for the practice of alternative and complementary medicine in California. He was also on the board of the California Homeopathic Medical Society and still edits the journal of this organization, the California Homeopath. He is the author of one book on the homeopathic study of tobacco and has written many articles for leading homeopathic journals, both in Europe and North America.

He has also spent over eight years traveling the world and has spent much of this time in India and parts of Africa. He has been involved in three different projects in Africa, including establishing a school in Ghana and working in an integrative medical clinic, and in Malawi he helped establish a homeopathic clinic in a rural part of the country. In Kenya he has been working with an existing homeopathy school, helping to establish a professional association and assisting in the educational development of students and graduates of the school. He has been working with homeopaths throughout the world, including Brazil, India, U.K, Australasia and North America.

The Natural Medicine Guide For Travel And Home

The Natural Medicine Guide For Travel And Home

Made in the USA
Charleston, SC
25 June 2013